Neuroembryology and Aging

Founded 2002 as 'Neuroembryology' by N. Ulfig, D.T.W. Yew and W.Y. Chan (2002–2005); Changed in 2005 to 'Neuroembryology and Aging'

KARGER

Printed in Switzerland on acid-free and non-aging paper (ISO 9706) by Reinhardt Druck, Basel

Appears quarterly: 1 volume per year (4 issues)

Neuroembryology and Aging

Guidelines for Authors

Types of Papers

The journal accepts the following types of papers: original papers, reviews, mini-reviews, short communications, case reports, technical reports, letters to the editor, commentaries and proceedings of meetings.

Submission

Only manuscripts written in English will be considered. They should be as concise as possible. Manuscripts should be submitted in triplicate (with three sets of illustrations of which one is an original; final high-resolution pictures need only be sent after acceptance of the paper) together with a soft copy on disc. For details, please refer to: www.karger.com/electronic_submission. The letter of submission should also be submitted at the same time to:

Professor Wood Yee Chan or
Professor David T.W. Yew
Editors-in-Chief
'Neuroembryology and Aging'
Department of Anatomy
Faculty of Medicine
The Chinese University of Hong Kong
Shatin, N.T. (Hong Kong)
Tel. +852 2609 6895
Fax +852 2603 5031
E-Mail: wy-chan@cuhk.edu.hk

Please adhere strictly to the instructions on style and arrangement (see 'Manuscript Preparation'); manuscripts which do not conform to the above are liable to be returned.

Papers must be accompanied by a cover letter including the names, phone and fax numbers of all authors, the complete address of the corresponding author, the title of the paper and a statement that the material has not been published and is not under current consideration for publication elsewhere. The letter must be signed by the corresponding author.

To make sure that papers are reviewed by suitable referees, authors should submit the name, address, fax number, e-mail address and field of interest of four candidate referees who are not directly concerned with the work being submitted. The Editor reserves the right to choose different referees from those suggested.

The Editors accept no responsibility for lost manuscripts. Authors should keep copies of everything submitted.

Papers describing studies on human subjects must include a statement that the studies were performed with the prior consent and understanding of both parents or legal guardians. Photographs of identifiable subjects must be accompanied by written permission for publication signed by both parents or legal guardians.

Manuscript Preparation

General

Authors may use UK or US spelling. All abbreviations must be written out in full when they first appear and the proposed abbreviation given in parentheses. Avoid using footnotes.

For judging the length of papers, the following estimation may be used:

- 3 typewritten (double-spaced) pages (with wide margins) = 1 printed page
- 800 words = 1 printed page
- title/author(s)/address(es)/abstract/key words = 0.75 printed pages
- 25 references = 0.5 printed pages

Title Page

The first page [3 typewritten (double-spaced) pages (with wide margins) = 1 printed page] of each paper should include:

- Title
- Authors' full names
- Institutional affiliations (with superscript letters that link them to the individual authors).

Example:
David T. Yew[a] Dietrich E. Lorke[b] Mang C. Yu[c]
Wood Yee Chan[a]

[a] Department of Anatomy, Facutly of Medicine, The Chinese University of Hong Kong, Hong Kong, China; [b] Department of Neuroanatomy, University of Hamburg, Hamburg, Germany; [c] Department of Anatomy and Cell Biology, University of Medicine and Dentistry of New Jersey, New Jersey Medical School, Newark, N.J., USA

- Short title for use as a running head (not in excess of 50 letter spaces)
- Full address of the corresponding author: exact postal address, phone and fax numbers, e-mail address

NB: Authors wishing to preserve the phonetic meaning of diacritics (PubMed reduces diacritics to their root characters) must spell their names accordingly when submitting manuscripts (e.g. Müller should be Mueller).

Original Papers

Original papers should include the following sections in the following sequence: Abstract, Key Words, Introduction, Materials and Methods, Results, Discussion, Acknowledgements, References.

Abstract: The abstract should summarize the essential new information contained in the paper; it should not exceed 200 words and should be structured as follows:

Background: What is the major problem that prompted the study?
Aims: What is the purpose of the study?
Results: Major findings, specific data.
Conclusions: Most important conclusions.
Avoid using abbreviations in the abstract.

Key Words: A list of 4–8 key words not appearing in the title should be provided.

Introduction: The objective of the study must be clearly stated. Sufficient background information, including relevant publications related to the study, should be outlined concisely. Extensive reviews of the literature should be avoided.

Materials and Methods: All the details necessary to reproduce the experiments must be included in this section. Ethically relevant aspects must be described in detail.

Results: In general, results should be presented descriptively (with minimal reference to earlier literature data or possible interpretations) and should be documented by photographs, schematic drawings (black and white), tables or diagrams. Tables and figures must be referred to in the text.

Discussion: First a brief summary of the major findings should be given without repeating parts of the 'Abstract' or of the 'Results' section. The results should be discussed in the context of relevant literature data. Extensive discussion and citations should be avoided.

Acknowledgements: Financial and material support, technical help and other assistance, and contributions which do not justify authorship should be acknowledged.

References

Cite references in the text using Arabic numerals [in square brackets]. Material submitted for publication but not yet accepted should be noted as 'unpublished data' and not be included in the reference list.

The list of references should include only those publications that are cited in the text. Do not alphabetize; number references in the order in which they are first mentioned in the text. The surnames of the authors followed by the initials should be given. There should be no punctuation other than commas to separate the authors. Preferably, please cite all authors. Abbreviate journal names according to the Index Medicus system. (Also see International Committee of Medical Journal Editors: Uniform requirements for manuscripts submitted to biomedical journals. N Engl J Med 1997;336: 309–315. www.icmje.org)

Authors are responsible for the accuracy of the references.

Digital Object Identifier (DOI)
S. Karger Publishers supports DOIs as unique identifiers for articles. A DOI number will be printed on the title page of each article. DOIs can be useful in the future for identifying and citing articles published online without volume or issue information. More information can be found at www.doi.org.

Examples
(a) Papers published in periodicals:
1 Chan WY, Lorke DE, Tiu SC, Yew DT: Proliferation and apoptosis in the developing human neocortex. Anat Rec 2002; 267:261-276.
(b) Papers published only with DOI numbers:
1 Theoharides TC, Boucher W, Spear K: Serum interleukin-6 reflects disease severity and osteoporosis in mastocytosis patients. Int Arch Allergy Immunol DOI: 10.1159/000063858.
(c) Monographs:
1 Matthews DE, Farewell VT: Using and Understanding Medical Statistics, ed 3. Basel, Karger, 1996.
(d) Edited books:
1 Kraig RP, Lascola CD, Caggiano A: Glial response to brain ischemia; in Kettenmann H, Ransom BR (eds): Neuroglia. Oxford, Oxford University Press, 1995, pp 964–976.

Reviews and All Other Types of Papers

Reviews: Reviews should be surveys and critical interpretations of recent research and concepts in the fields covered by the journal. An abstract and key words are required. There are no restrictions on the number of pages or illustrations.

Mini-Reviews: Mini-reviews on topics of particular current interest are considered. Mini-reviews should normally not exceed 7 printed pages. An abstract and key words (see 'Original Papers') are required. Manuscripts can be divided into sections at the author's discretion.

Short Communications: Short communications should not exceed 2–4 printed pages. No preliminary findings should be reported. Only short but complete (in all aspects) reports of studies can be accepted. Short communications do not need any section headings. An abstract (not exceeding 70 words) and 4–6 key words are required.

KARGER

Fax +41 61 306 12 34
E-Mail karger@karger.ch
www.karger.com

The Guidelines for Authors are available at:
www.karger.com/nba_Guidelines

Case Reports: Case reports should describe new, noteworthy or unusual findings, or provide new insights into a problem. They should be divided into sections (see 'Original Papers'). The 'Results' and 'Discussion' sections may be combined. Four printed pages is the maximum for case reports. An abstract (not exceeding 70 words) and 4–6 key words are required.

Technical Reports: Technical reports describing novel methodological approaches associated with the fields of this journal are also encouraged. Full-length papers should be divided into sections (see 'Original Papers'). For accelerated publication, short technical reports may be submitted as 'Short Communications'.

Letters to the Editor: Letters should comment on papers previously published in this journal or on a topic of current interest. They should not exceed 500 words and should be accompanied by up to 10 references but no illustrations. Neither abstracts nor key words are required.

Commentaries: Commentaries should express an opinion/viewpoint or hypothesis on a current topic of neuroembryology and aging. They should not exceed 3 printed pages, including 1 illustration and 10–15 references.

Proceedings of Meetings: Full papers or abstracts of material presented at scientific meetings can be published at the discretion of the Editor.

Illustrations and Tables

Illustrations prepared on separate sheets must be in a finished form, ready for reproduction.

Tables require a heading and figures a legend.

Well-contrasted photographic prints, trimmed at right angles and in the final size are required.

If possible, group several illustrations on one plate for reproduction.

Figures should be provided ready for 'same-size' reproduction; they must correspond in size with either a single-column width (8.8 cm) or double-column width (18.0 cm). The maximal length is 22.3 cm. Line drawings should be submitted in their final size.

Computer drawings will be accepted provided they are of a quality comparable with line drawings. Lines and curves must be smooth.

Any lettering, pointers or scale bars should be applied directly to the illustrations using Letraset or similar adhesive labels. Letters should be 3 mm in height and may be white or outlined in white when placed on a dark background. Magnifications should be indicated by scale bars on the figures.

Indicate the figure number, the first author's name, and the proper orientation (e.g. 'top') on the back of each illustration.

Electronically submitted b/w half-tone and color illustrations must have a final resolution of 300 dpi after scaling, line drawings one of 800–1,200 dpi.

In general, the same data should not be presented in both figure and table form.

Figures should be referred to in the text as (fig. 10) or figure 10.

Copyright, Proofs, Reprints

Submission of an article for publication implies the transfer of the copyright from the author(s) to the publisher upon acceptance. All accepted manuscripts become the permanent property of 'Neuroembryology and Aging' and may not be published elsewhere, in whole or in part, without the written consent of the publisher. It is the (corresponding) author's responsibility to obtain permission to reproduce illustrations or tables from other publications.

Manuscripts, disks and illustrations will not be returned. Authors wishing the return of original illustrations should state so.

Proofs will be sent to the corresponding author and should be returned with the least possible delay (normally within 3 days). Alterations made in proofs, other than the correction of printer's errors, are charged to the corresponding author.

Author's Choice™

With this option the author can choose to make his article freely available online against a one-time fee of CHF 2750.–. This fee is independent of any standard charges for supplementary pages, color images etc. which may apply. More information can be found at www.karger.com/authors_choice.

General Information

Neuroembryology and Aging

ISSN Print Edition: 1661–3406
ISSN Online Edition: 1661–3414

Journal Homepage: www.karger.com/nba

Publication Data: 'Neuroembryology and Aging' is published 4 times a year. Volume 5 with 4 issues appears in 2008.

Subscription Rates: Subscriptions run for a full calendar year. Prices are given per year.

Personal subscription:

Print or Online	Print+Online combined
CHF 380.–	CHF 425.–
EUR 271.50	EUR 303.50
USD 345.50	USD 386.50

postage and handling (added to print and print+online)
CHF 24.– Europe, CHF 36.– Overseas
EUR 17.20
USD 33.00

Institutional subscription:

Print or Online	Print+Online combined
CHF 760.–	CHF 836.–
EUR 543.–	EUR 597.–
USD 691.00	USD 760.00

postage and handling (added to print and print+online)
CHF 30.– Europe, CHF 45.– Overseas
EUR 21.60
USD 41.20

Airmail surcharge: CHF 30.40 / USD 27.60

Back Volumes and Single Issues: Information on availability and prices of single print issues and print or electronic back volumes can be obtained from Customer Service at *service@karger.ch.*

Bibliographic Indices: This journal is regularly listed in bibliographic services, including *Current Contents*® and PubMed/MEDLINE.

Photocopying: This journal has been registered with the Copyright Clearance Center (CCC), as indicated by the code appearing on the first page of each article. For readers in the US, this code signals consent for copying of articles for personal or internal use, or for the personal or internal use of specific clients, provided that the stated fee is paid per copy directly to
Copyright Clearance Center Inc.
222 Rosewood Drive
Danvers, MA 01923 (USA)
A copy of the first page of the article must accompany payment. Consent does not extend to copying for general distribution, for promotion, for creating new works, or for resale. In these cases, specific written permission must be obtained from the copyright owner,
S. Karger AG, P.O. Box
CH–4009 Basel (Switzerland).

Subscription Orders:
Orders can be placed at agencies, bookstores, directly with the Publisher or further Karger offices or representatives:

S. Karger AG
Medical and Scientific Publishers
P.O. Box
CH–4009 Basel
Switzerland
(for courier services only:
Allschwilerstrasse 10
CH–4055 Basel)
Tel. +41 61 306 11 11
Fax +41 61 306 12 34
E-Mail karger@karger.ch
www.karger.com

France:
Librairie Medi-Sciences Sarl
36, bd de Latour-Maubourg
75007 Paris
France
Tél. +33 (0) 1 45 51 42 58
Fax +33 (0) 1 45 56 07 80
E-Mail librairie@medi-sciences.fr
www.medi-sciences.fr

Germany:
S. Karger GmbH
Postfach
79095 Freiburg
Deutschland
(Hausadresse: Lörracher Strasse 16A
79115 Freiburg)
Tel. +49 761 45 20 70
Fax +49 761 45 20 714
E-Post information@karger.de
www.karger.de

India, Bangladesh, Sri Lanka:
Panther Publishers Private Ltd.
33, First Main
Koramangala First Block
Bangalore 560 034
India
Tel. +91 80 25505 836
Tel. +91 80 25505 837
Fax +91 80 25505 981
E-Mail panther_publishers@vsnl.com
www.pantherpublishers.com

Japan:
Karger Japan, Inc.
Yushima S Bld. 3F
4-2-3, Yushima, Bunkyo-ku
Tokyo 113-0034
Japan
Tel. +81 3 3815 1800
Fax +81 3 3815 1802
E-Mail publisher@karger.jp

China, Taiwan and Malaysia:
Karger China
Suite 409, Apollo Building
1440 Central Yan An Road
Shanghai 200040
China
Tel. +86-21-6133 1861
Fax +86-21-6133 1862
E-Mail karger.ray@gmail.com

South America and Central America:
Cranbury International LLC
7 Clarendon Ave., Suite 2
Montpelier, VT 05602
USA
Tel. +1 802 223 6565
Fax +1 802 223 6824
E-Mail
eatkin@cranburyinternational.com
www.cranburyinternational.com

United Kingdom, Ireland:
S. Karger AG
c/o London Liaison Office
4 Rickett Street
London SW6 1RU
United Kingdom
Tel. +44 (0) 20 7386 0500
Fax +44 (0) 20 7610 3337
E-Mail uk@karger.ch

USA:
S. Karger Publishers, Inc.
26 West Avon Road
P.O. Box 529
Unionville, CT 06085
USA
Toll free: +1 800 828 5479
Tel. +1 860 675-7834
Fax +1 860 675-7302
E-Mail karger@snet.net

Change of Address:
Both old and new address should be sent to the subscription source.

KARGER

Fax +41 61 306 12 34
E-Mail karger@karger.ch
www.karger.com

The Journal Home Page is available at:
www.karger.com/nba

The first book to provide a truly comprehensive perspective

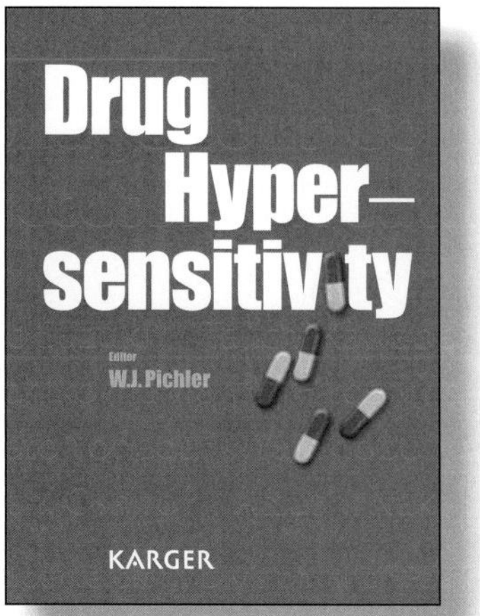

Drug Hypersensitivity

Editor
Werner J. Pichler

Allergy, Pharmacology, Immunology, Dermatology, Toxicology, Metabolism, Hepatology, Nephrology, General Medicine

Contents

www.karger.com/drug_hypersensitivity

KI 07227

Drug Hypersensitivity
Editor: Pichler, W.J. (Bern)
X + 438 p., 78 fig., 58 in color, 78 tab., hard cover, 2007
CHF 274.– / EUR 195.50 / USD 274.00
Prices subject to change
EUR price for Germany, USD price for USA only
ISBN 978-3-8055-8269-8

KARGER

Order Form

Please send: ______ copy/ies
Postage and handling free with prepayment

Payment:
Please charge to my credit card
☐ American Express ☐ Diners ☐ Eurocard
☐ MasterCard ☐ Visa

Card No.: ______________________
Exp. date: ______________________
CVV/CVC ______________________
(3 digits in the signature field on the back of VISA and Mastercard)

☐ Check enclosed ☐ Please bill me

Orders may be placed with any bookshop, subscription agency, directly with the publisher or through a Karger distributor.

Fax: +41 61 306 12 34
S. Karger AG, P.O. Box, CH–4009 Basel (Switzerland)
E-Mail orders@karger.ch, **www.karger.com**

Name/Address: ______________________

Date: ______________________

Signature: ______________________

Neuroembryology and Aging

Obituary

It is our sad duty to inform you that our son Steven Karger passed away on March 5, 2008. Surrounded by his family, he died peacefully, exhausted after his long and intense battle against brain cancer.

Born in 1959 as our eldest son, he joined the family business in 1982. After his studies in marketing and economics, Steven chose to learn and hone the skills of his trade directly on the job, first as an intern with other publishers, then as my right hand, and later as managing director of the bookshop and agency Karger Libri as well as the German branch of our publishing business. As of July 1999, Steven held the position of CEO and was responsible for the day-to-day business of all Karger enterprises worldwide.

With his openness, warmth and abundance of energy, he led the company successfully into the new millennium and the electronic era, his leadership being characterized by respect, honesty, caring and a wonderful sense of humor. The values and principles guiding him throughout his life were securely anchored in his religious faith, tradition and heritage. His keen interest in people and the world around him led him to seek out innovations and at the same time maintain company values such as quality, independence and good customer service.

Steven Karger was a loving family man and leaves a wife and three children. He was a wonderful and reliable friend. He was involved in many cultural and social activities and projects in his city and community and was well known as someone who would generously contribute both his personal time and energy for a good cause. As an amateur flutist in the best sense of the word, he always found classical music to be a source of strength, solace and inspiration.

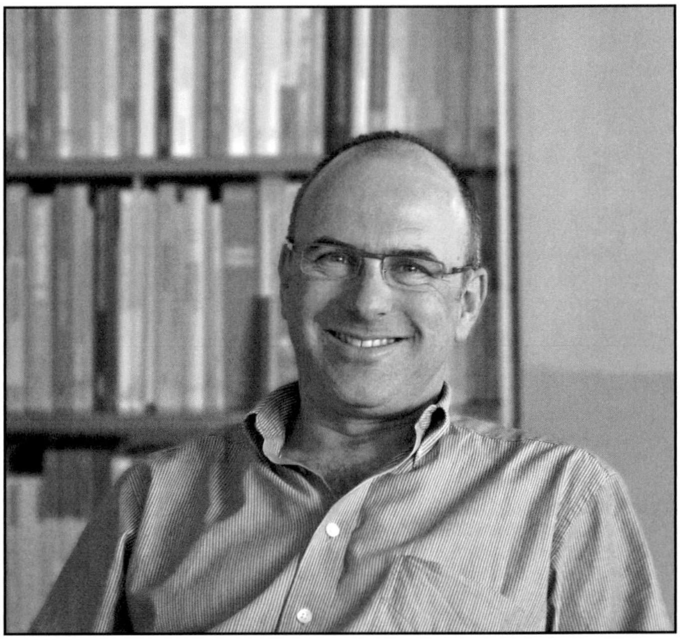

Steven Karger (1959–2008)

He touched many lives and will be remembered not only for his astute business knowledge but mostly for his sincere, warm and caring nature.

Our youngest daughter Gabriella Karger will be taking over his business responsibilities.

Thomas and Yvette Karger and family

KARGER
Fax +41 61 306 12 34
E-Mail karger@karger.ch
www.karger.com

Thomas Karger
S. Karger Publishers
Allschwilerstrasse 10
4055 Basel (Switzerland)

Neuroembryology and Aging

Imaging of the Developing Brain

Editors
David T.W. Yew, Hong Kong
Wood Yee Chan, Hong Kong

52 figures, 7 in color, and 3 tables, 2008

KARGER
Basel · Freiburg · Paris · London · New York · Bangalore · Bangkok · Shanghai · Singapore · Tokyo · Sydney

S. Karger
Medical and Scientific Publishers
Basel • Freiburg • Paris • London
New York • Bangalore • Bangkok
Shanghai • Singapore • Tokyo • Sydney

Disclaimer
The statements, options and data contained in this publication are solely those of the individual authors and contributors and not of the publisher and the editor(s). The appearance of advertisements in the journal is not a warranty, endorsement, or approval of the products or services advertised or of their effectiveness, quality or safety. The publisher and the editor(s) disclaim responsibility for any injury to persons or property resulting from any ideas, methods, instructions or products referred to in the content or advertisements.

Drug Dosage
The authors and the publisher have exerted every effort to ensure that drug selection and dosage set forth in this text are in accord with current recommendations and practice at the time of publication. However, in view of ongoing research, changes in government regulations, and the constant flow of information relating to drug therapy and drug reactions, the reader is urged to check the package insert for each drug for any change in indications and dosage and for added warnings and precautions. This is particularly important when the recommended agent is a new and/or infrequently employed drug.

Printed in Switzerland
on acid-free and non-aging paper (ISO 9706) by
Reinhardt Druck, Basel
ISBN 978–3–8055–8546–0

KARGER

Fax +41 61 306 12 34
E-Mail karger@karger.ch
www.karger.com

Neuroembryology and Aging

Vol. 5, No. 1–2, 2008

Contents

KARGER

Fax +41 61 306 12 34
E-Mail karger@karger.ch
www.karger.com

Access to full text and tables of contents, including tentative ones for forthcoming issues:
www.karger.com/nba_issues

Neuroembryology and Aging

Neuroembryol Aging 2008;5:5
DOI: 10.1159/000116726

Published online: August 19, 2008

Editorial

Magnetic resonance imaging (MRI), ultrasound and angiography are all important imaging techniques that medical science has begun to employ extensively in the human in the last few decades. Their uses in studies of the developing nervous system, however, still have some limitations despite the continually improving design of the technology. In this volume, we present reviews as well as new findings on the usage of these techniques in the fetal and neonatal human and in animal models. Papers in this volume review aspects of normal development [Xu et al.; Yang et al.; Ying et al.] as well as abnormal changes [Tao and Yew; Ying et al.]. The basics of MRI are elucidated in a short review by Shi et al., including examples of functional MRI (fMRI) studies in animals. The review by Wilke and Holland presents the issues and opportunities of MRI. Another review by Antonio et al. outlines various types of MRI techniques and demonstrates that MRI can be used to decipher the complexities of neuronal pathways, thus solving the greatest difficulties for anatomists in the past: serial sections and reconstruction. Two papers review nervous system malformations [Salman; Tao and Yew], which will likely be further explored extensively by imaging in the days to come. Functional MRI on both human and animal nervous systems is reviewed by other papers in this volume, with particular focus on the developmental stages.

It is hoped that this volume will prove useful to further the interest of scientists and physicians actively engaged in the field, and arouse the curiosity of those embarking on the research and clinical applications which are now made possible by MRI, ultrasound and angiography.

D.T. Yew
W.Y. Chan

KARGER

Fax +41 61 306 12 34
E-Mail karger@karger.ch
www.karger.com

1661–3406/08/0052–0005$24.50/0

Accessible online at:
www.karger.com/nba

Neuroembryology and Aging

Neuroembryol Aging 2008;5:6–13
DOI: 10.1159/000116727

Received: March 27, 2007
Accepted: June 12, 2007
Published online: August 19, 2008

Structural MR Imaging Studies of the Brain in Children: Issues and Opportunities

Marko Wilke[a, b] Scott K. Holland[c]

[a]Pediatric Neurology and Developmental Medicine, Children's Hospital, and [b]Section of Experimental MR of the CNS, Department of Neuroradiology, University of Tübingen, Tübingen, Germany; [c]Imaging Research Center, Cincinnati Children's Hospital Medical Center, Cincinnati, Ohio, USA

Key Words

Data acquisition · Head coil size · Magnetic resonance imaging · Neuroimaging studies in children · Pediatric imaging · Reference data

Abstract

Structural magnetic resonance imaging has gained widespread attention over the last decade, especially following the advances in automated image processing algorithms. It is an interesting approach that, among other applications, allows investigating and describing normal and disturbed human brain development. With this overview, we aim to point out special aspects that may arise when imaging children, with regard to study design, data acquisition and data processing. We conclude with shortly addressing the potential insights to be gained from such studies.

Introduction

Before non-invasive neuroimaging methods were widely available, knowledge about normal brain development was surprisingly scarce [1], as the classical approach, postmortem neuroanatomical studies, was limited by the low mortality of normal children [2]. Following the introduction of computed tomography and positron emission tomography, first attempts to describe brain development were made [3]. However, these techniques invariably expose the subject to ionizing radiation, which makes them unsuitable for studying truly normal children due to ethical concerns. It was therefore only after the introduction of magnetic resonance imaging (MRI) that normal brain development could be assessed in a more systematic fashion. The technique gives excellent soft tissue contrast, is repeatable and has become more and more widely available. Consequently, normal brain development has been the focus of a growing number of MRI studies in the past [2, 4–12].

However, children are not small adults, and imaging children presents a number of special challenges on several levels [13]. In this review, we would therefore like to highlight several issues that may need to be taken into account when planning and conducting structural MRI studies involving children. We do not aim at exhaustively covering all aspects of neuroimaging that might differ between studies in pediatric and adult subjects. Instead, we will present a rather selective list of possible issues that are likely to arise, based on our experience and assess-

KARGER

Fax +41 61 306 12 34
E-Mail karger@karger.ch
www.karger.com

1661–3406/08/0052–0006$24.50/0

Accessible online at:
www.karger.com/nba

Marko Wilke, MD, Department of Pediatric Neurology and Developmental Medicine
Children's Hospital, University of Tübingen, Hoppe Seyler Street 1
DE–72076 Tübingen (Germany)
Tel. +49 7071 29 83416, Fax +49 7071 29 5473
E-Mail Marko.Wilke@med.uni-tuebingen.de

Table 1. Overview of points raised in this paper

Study design issues	Data acquisition issues	Data processing issues	Data analysis issues
Ethical requirements	Technical issues	Spatial normalization	Narrow age range
Dealing with incidental findings	Optimized sequences	Adequate reference data	Manual or automated processing
Adequate group sizes	Adequate coils	Tissue segmentation	Carefully defined groups
Truly normal controls	Scanning time	Adequate reference data	Nuisance variables
Personal history	Practical issues	Prior-less approach	
Family history	Preparation scheme		
Neuropsychological and handedness assessment	Mock scanner		
	Motivated personnel		
	Adequate time slots		
	Distraction		

ment in this field. The following main points will be addressed: issues of study design, data acquisition, data processing and data analysis (table 1). Lastly, we will try to provide an outlook as to where such studies will lead us and what kind of insights may be gained.

Study Design Issues

There are a number of special considerations when planning pediatric neuroimaging studies. First, it is imperative that pediatric research protocols adhere to the strictest ethical standards. Accordingly, *institutional review boards* can be expected to scrutinize medical research protocols involving children. The issue of informed consent of a minor presents a special ethical dilemma for the investigator and institutional review board alike and therefore neuroimaging studies involving children under the age of 18 years must meet the highest ethical standards [14]. This includes the necessity to assess the available scans for the presence of *incidental findings* [15], which, although rare, do occur at a rate of 2% typically and pose a special problem in a healthy population [16, 17]. The National Institutes of Health in the USA have made a recommendation of full disclosure of incidental findings as well as for establishing a mechanism for reporting such findings to subjects and their physicians [18].

Power analyses and *group size* calculations for pediatric neuroimaging studies should allow for higher failure rates especially among younger children [19]. Moreover, the high variability in brain structures in children [20, 21] will make the detection of subtle differences in brain structure and function with age very difficult when only small sample sizes are used. When aiming to study *'normal children'*, several studies have shown that imaging data from children acquired during a clinically indicated examination is not equivalent to imaging data from truly normal children recruited from the community [22, 23]. In special cases, such data may not be available due to ethical concerns (e.g. imaging toddlers which would require sedation [24]). Under such circumstances, there may be no other choice than to recruit 'normal' subjects from clinical populations. However, in this case images should be carefully reviewed by qualified radiologists or other imaging specialists, to rule out abnormalities and exclude data sets where pathology is found. Furthermore, especially disorders with a putative neurodevelopmental background like attention deficit/hyperactivity disorder (ADHD) or schizophrenia have been shown to present a spectrum of abnormalities, parts of which are also present in clinically unaffected first-degree relatives [25, 26]. It is therefore prudent to consider *family history* when recruiting subjects, as well as *previous events* potentially interfering with normal brain development, like premature birth, significant head trauma, or other neurologic or neuropsychiatric diseases.

Assessing and reporting *handedness* of study populations should be standard practice, due to the known influence on brain structure [27]. However, the optimal method for characterizing handedness is still controversial. While many researchers use simple questionnaires like the Edinburgh Handedness Inventory [28], others prefer more elaborate tests involving actual performance testing (like the hand dominance test [29]). In our opinion, if handedness is not critical to the study question at hand, a questionnaire approach is sufficient (provided the child is not left alone in filling it out), especially as the results from such manual performance tests have been shown to be strongly correlated with data collected using

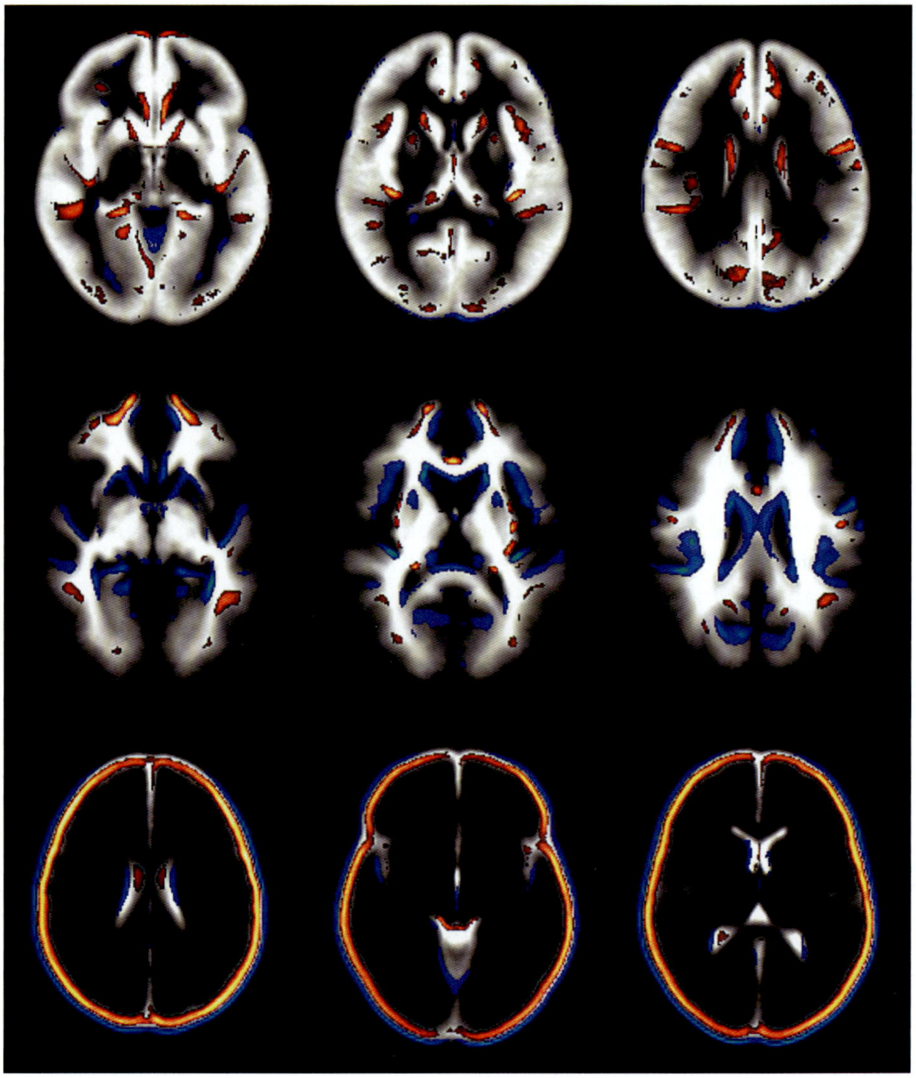

Fig. 1. Tissue concentration differences (>20%) for gray matter, white matter and cerebrospinal fluid between pediatric and adult reference data. Data from 200 normal children [21] were compared with the Montreal Neurological Institute standard adult template [36]: red: higher density in children; blue: higher density in adults; children have proportionally more gray matter, but less white matter and CSF.

the Edinburgh Handedness Inventory [30]. For studies aiming to investigate the structural basis of cognitive functions in a broader sense, a *neuropsychological assessment* of each participant seems warranted, potentially with special emphasis on the function focused on (e.g. language or working memory).

Data Acquisition Issues

Data acquisition presents several technical challenges and practical difficulties. On the *technical* side, the brain of a child has a different tissue composition (fig. 1) and water content, and *sequences* may have to be adapted accordingly. For example, three different optimized TR/TE combinations for spin echo sequences have been suggested for use in the 1st year of life alone [3]. For very small baby heads, the *coil* design may become an issue. Ideally, the radiofrequency head coil should be optimally fitted to the size of the head being examined. Therefore, infant brain images acquired in an adult head coil will suffer from somewhat suboptimal signal-to-noise ratios due to poor coil loading compared to what would be possible with a smaller-diameter head coil designed specifically for smaller heads. Extremity coils have been used as alternatives [31]. Recently, MR-compatible incubators have been introduced that allow a much more considerate approach to imaging [32] (fig. 2). While such scans will still likely be done mainly for clinical purposes, studies (for example investigating the effects of prematurity [33]) obtained as a byproduct of a clinically indicated scan are made much easier by such custom-tailored solutions. However, the infrastructural requirements are intensive and expensive.

In pediatric imaging, the need to balance the highest-attainable data quality with *time constraints* is much more pressing than when imaging adults. Particularly in the context of an add-on to a clinically indicated imaging study it may be necessary to minimize the time required for the research scanning protocol in order to be more child-friendly in terms of simply not taking too long [3, 13]. For example, a 30-min anatomical scan may yield superior signal-to-noise and spatial resolution but will be spoiled by motion artifacts in such a high subset of children that a shorter version would provide an overall higher yield in terms of usable data.

Practical issues arise from the high degree of compliance necessary to participate in an imaging study. Children experience less claustrophobia, but fear and the lack of abstract understanding of 'what is going on' are major issues [13, 19]. Considering the age when children are able to meet these high demands, surprisingly the first few months of life offer a window of opportunity because newborns tend to go to sleep predictably after nursing, which can be used to acquire images during natural sleep [34]. However, for the following years (1–4 years of age, which are most interesting with regard to the enormous developmental progress children make during these years), it is nearly impossible to do MRI studies in healthy and awake children. In this case, one can wait hopefully for the child to fall asleep in the scanner [11], but this may take a long time due to the excitement and is likely to result in a high failure rate. Experienced researchers start to include children in scientific studies when they reach 5–6 years of age, which is when most children are able to remain still over the periods of time necessary to acquire an image [19]. In our experience, the *preparation* of children is critical to establishing trust and to ensure at least the willingness to cooperate (if not necessarily the ability [13]). To this effect, custom-made introductory videos or life-sized dolls (being imaged before the child; fig. 3) have proven to be effective in alleviating the tension. The use of *mock scanners* has been advocated by some researchers [35], but in our experience is not a necessary prerequisite for successful large-scale studies. However, children may benefit from such desensitization, so especially if time is not readily available on the 'real' MRI scanner for this purpose, the mock scanner can be a cost-effective alternative. Overall, even with an extensive preparation routine, about 50% of children in the very young age group will fail the first attempt [19]. Last but not least, the *personnel* conducting the actual examination involving children must be willing to accommodate a child's individual needs for explanations, e.g. to provide the time to get accustomed to the situation. A calm and child-centered atmosphere around the scanner therefore is an obvious necessity, and enough *time* must be available by reserving longer-than-usual slots for brain scans in children. During scanning, maximum comfort must be ensured and ideally, *distraction* in the form of music or even video entertainment should be available.

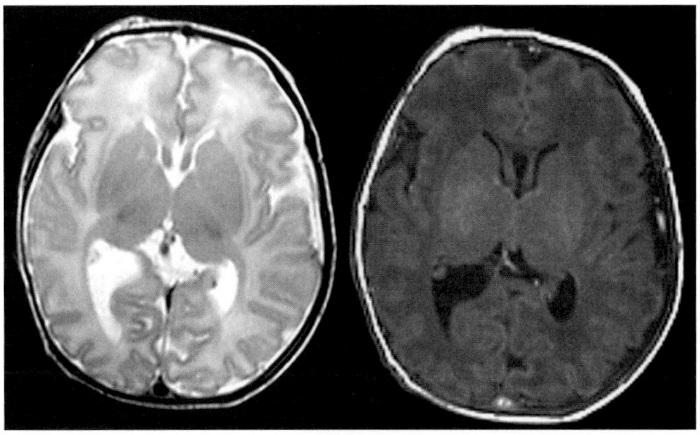

Fig. 2. Axial T_2-weighted (left) and corresponding T_1-weighted (right) image from a premature infant acquired using an MR-compatible incubator. Note high image quality.

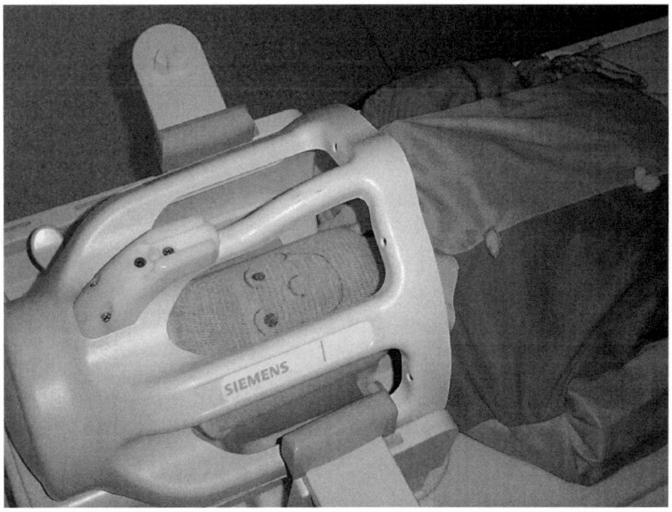

Color version available online

Fig. 3. Life-sized doll (dressed in a clown's costume) in the actual MR scanner, alleviating fear and discomfort especially in younger children.

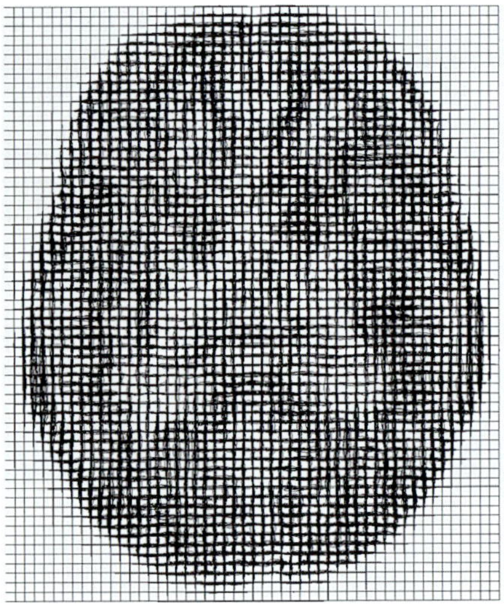

Fig. 4. Deformations resulting from warping the brain of a 7-year-old child to an adult template, illustrating the regional differences between the two images which are due to the non-linear aspects of spatial normalization (axial slice, ±20 mm from the anterior commissure). Note strong deformation occurring all over the cortical gray matter.

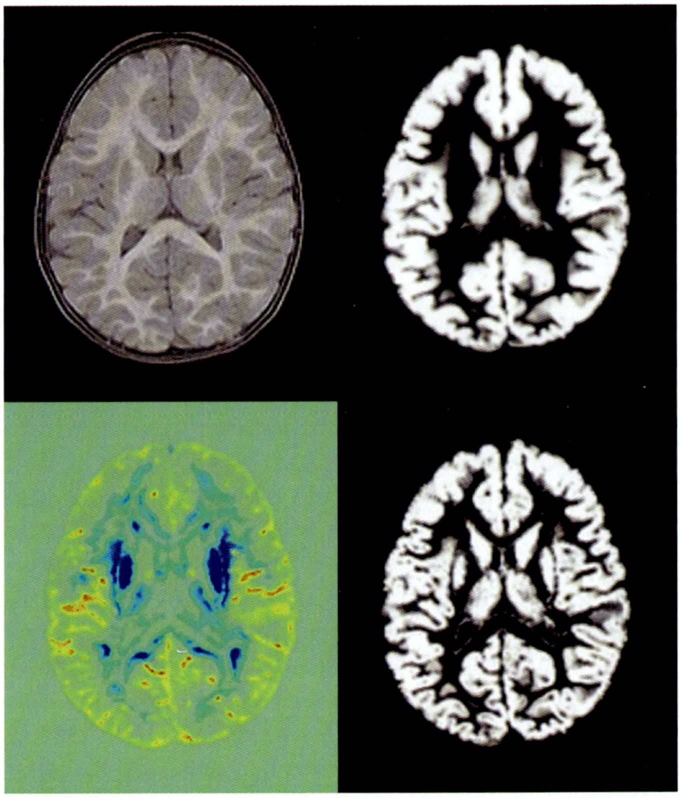

Fig. 5. Results from processing a neonatal brain image (left): the standard approach (top) [41] results in serious tissue misclassification; an optimized approach (bottom) involving a neonatal template for normalization and not using tissue priors for segmentation [57] yields much more realistic results; bottom left: difference image.

Data Processing Issues

Obviously, a data processing approach that was developed using adult data and that makes any kind of assumptions about the properties of data acquired from children is prone to be wrong with these assumptions (fig. 1, 4). Assumptions that cast the pediatric brain as a small adult brain for imaging purposes become increasingly erroneous with the age difference between the subject group of interest and the data being used for reference. For example, brain size, shape and tissue composition may not differ substantially between a 17-year-old teenager and a 20-year-old young adult. However, the brain of a 6-year-old has been shown to have different proportions, tissue composition and relative structure sizes (e.g. larger basal ganglia or more prominent parietal lobes) when compared with adult reference data [4, 7, 8], and a newborn's brain is entirely different again [33]. It should be noted that the problem goes 'both ways' as most reference data have been compiled using healthy young subjects; for example, the widely used brain template from the Montreal Neurological Institute consists of subjects with a mean age of 26 years [36]. Therefore, not only subjects significantly younger but also substantially older (e.g. studies involving patients with Alzheimer disease) will be processed based on inappropriate reference data.

In the case of image data processing, two crucial steps we examined earlier are *spatial normalization* and *tissue segmentation* [37, 38] (fig. 1, 4). Both are necessary steps in structural image data processing in group analyses. Spatial normalization, aimed at removing differences between images with regard to orientation, shape and size [39, 40], is prone to do injustice to brain regions that differ the most from the subject(s) contributing to the reference frame. In the case of children's brains, this mainly includes the parietal lobe and the basal ganglia where pediatric brain imaging data must be severely distorted in order to match the adult reference frame [4, 7, 37]. Such distortions will mainly be introduced if matching on the regional level is chosen (i.e. a non-linear transformation [40]). The global scaling resulting from a purely linear, affine-only normalization has been shown to not correlate significantly with age (in the age range of 5–18 years of age [37]). Tissue segmentation relies on two main approaches to identify tissue classes (typically gray matter, white matter, cerebrospinal fluid and non-brain tissue) in one image: (1) intensity information ('does it have the intensity of gray matter?') and (2) spatial information ('is it where I expect gray matter?'). Modern algorithms for brain imaging segmentation combine the information from both approaches in very complex ways [41]. For either approach, prior knowledge in some form must be passed to the algorithm in order to allow for a classification. In both cases, the assumptions based on adult data are violated in pediatric imaging data: especially in younger children, unmyelinated white matter constitutes a tissue class that is not present in adults [33, 42], and the spatial distribution of brain tissue classes (and their relation to each other) is substantially different between children and adults [38] (fig. 1). Consequently, appropriate reference data must be used especially when dealing with data from younger subjects. Alternatively (or additionally), approaches that do not heavily rely on such reference information may be preferable in segmenting images from an age group for which adequate prior probability information is not available. An example of segmentation of an infant brain image using adult spatial reference information (prior probability tissue maps) or without such information (relying on tissue intensity alone) illustrates this point in figure 5.

Data Analysis Issues

What was said above is also relevant for data analysis: the developing brain is a moving target, continuously undergoing changes on different levels [2, 4–2], being most relevant for brain image analysis. There are significant differences in the brain image characteristics of a toddler, a 10-year-old, and a 16-year-old. This implies that, in cross-sectional imaging studies not aimed at investigating the effect of aging, the age range of subjects included should be as narrow as possible. Only thus can the confounding effects of changes accompanying normal brain development be minimized [43]. Otherwise processing steps adequate for the one extreme will be inadequate for the other end of the age span and vice versa. Also, even if all brains are processed correctly, the inherent increase in variability induced by developmental changes [20, 21] will decrease the likelihood to detect similarities within such a group.

Approaches to anatomical image analysis can be divided into manual methods and automated *analysis approaches* [44, 45]. As in the case of adult imaging data, there are arguments in favor of each approach. A careful manual delineation by a neuroanatomically trained rater will, in a single case, likely yield better results than an automated labeling approach (especially in hard-to-segment smaller structures like the amygdala or the thalamus [46]). However, these tracings are extremely laborious and time-consuming procedures and thus effectively prohibit the assessment of the larger sample sizes called for in pediatric structural neuroimaging studies as detailed above [12, 23]. In our experience, methodologically adapted automated procedures that are able to assess larger groups and allow for later voxel-based or regional analyses are most effective. However, this choice is mainly a function of the question at hand; the available data, possible algorithms and, of course, manpower also need to be considered. Overall, there is no simple answer to this question, especially as results from both approaches may be complementary [47, 48].

With regard to the increasing tendency to relate measures of cortical thickness, local or regional tissue volume or other structural measures to external variables (e.g. IQ, gender or disease status [49–52]), great care must be taken to avoid interdependencies with possibly confounding factors. For example, a typical clinical sample of subjects with ADHD will contain a number of subjects showing comorbid obsessive-compulsive disorder (OCD) [53]. Comparisons involving such a sample and a healthy control group may be able to identify regions of shared pathology (between ADHD and OCD) and profound differences (between ADHD and/or OCD and controls), but will be unable to identify specifically the neuroanatomical substrate of ADHD alone (if there is one) [54]. Variability due to the mixed pathology may make the detection of smaller effects impossible, or worse, their effects will dominate the results; particularly when age is included as another variable. Therefore, a well-designed neuroimaging study must carefully *characterize* subjects using detailed inclusion and exclusion criteria. During the data analysis process *nuisance variables* of known influence on brain structure should be incorporated in the statistical model as covariates and accounted for. Especially with younger children, we tend to use age in months (as opposed to years), handedness, gender and IQ (or, if not available, years of parental education [55]) as covariates; further variables will be considered depending on the question at hand [6, 43, 56]. Of course, strong correlations between variables (e.g. all controls are right-handed while all patients are left-handed) cannot be accounted for. As noted above, the normal structural variability inherent even in 'homogenous' groups of children [20, 21] calls for large samples to begin with.

Conclusion and Outlook

Children are not simply small adults. This is true in sickness and in health for MRI studies. As elaborated above, study design, acquisition, processing, and analysis call for special consideration. For example, a child may not be able to remain still for 20 min (or substantially longer) for a brain imaging study, and our tools to process MRI data have been developed and optimized based on adult data which may not be adequate for pediatric imaging data. The added complexity in pediatric imaging studies calls for an analogous complexity in the team required to perform them: radiological, pediatric and image processing skills must be combined in order to successfully execute such studies.

There are a number of possible implications that structural MRI studies may have in the future: for one, classification schemes based on clinical information may profit from a more biologically founded approach, allowing to further define diseases based on subtle neuroanatomical differences. The identification of such predictors would enhance our understanding of the biological underpinning of neurological or neurodevelopmental disorders. Ultimately, treatment-response-predicting changes would be most valuable clinically.

It should be stated that, although knowing 'where' is not equivalent to understanding 'why', such location information may allow to detect certain parallels and could guide the choice of complementary methods. It is therefore tempting to speculate on how (simple or complicated) structure-function relationships could advance our understanding of neurological disorders. Finally, understanding normal development and the influence of adverse factors might allow for earlier and more targeted interventions. To conclude, we believe that a wide range of questions in the field of developmental neuroimaging is still open for discussion, and structural MRI studies may be one of our tools to address them.

Acknowledgments

This work was funded in part by the German Research Council, DFG-SFB 550, C4, and by a grant from the National Institutes of Child Health and Human Development, RO1-HD38578. We are indebted to Ingeborg Krägeloh-Mann, MD, PhD, and Wolfgang Grodd, MD, PhD, for continued support. We would also like to thank Thomas Naegele, MD, PhD, Wolfgang Grodd, MD, PhD, and Christian Gaser, PhD, for supplying figure material (fig. 2, 3 and 5, respectively).

References

1 Giedd JN, Snell JW, Lange N, Rajapakse JC, Casey BJ, Kozuch PL, Vaituzis AC, Vauss YC, Hamburger SD, Kaysen D, Rapoport JL: Quantitative magnetic resonance imaging of human brain development: ages 4–18. Cereb Cortex 1996;6:551–560.

2 Courchesne E, Chisum HJ, Townsend J, Cowles A, Covington J, Egaas B, Harwood M, Hinds S, Press GA: Normal brain development and aging: quantitative analysis at in vivo MR imaging in healthy volunteers. Radiology 2000;216:672–682.

3 Ball WS Jr, Dunn RS: Computed tomography and magnetic resonance imaging; in Ball WS Jr (ed): Pediatric Neuroradiology, ed 1. Philadelphia, Lippincott Raven, 1997, p 17.

4 Sowell ER, Thompson PM, Holmes CJ, Batth R, Jernigan TL, Toga AW: Localizing age-related changes in brain structure between childhood and adolescence using statistical parametric mapping. Neuroimage 1999;9:587–597.

5 Pfefferbaum A, Mathalon DH, Sullivan EV, Rawles JM, Zipursky RB, Lim KO: A quantitative magnetic resonance imaging study of changes in brain morphology from infancy to late adulthood. Arch Neurol 1994;51:874–887.

6 Reiss AL, Abrams MT, Singer HS, Ross JL, Denckla MB: Brain development, gender and IQ in children. A volumetric imaging study. Brain 1996;119:1763–1774.

7 Giedd JN, Blumenthal J, Jeffries NO, Castellanos FX, Liu H, Zijdenbos A, Paus T, Evans AC, Rapoport JL: Brain development during childhood and adolescence: a longitudinal MRI study. Nat Neurosci 1999;2:861–863.

8 Castellanos FX, Lee PP, Sharp W, Jeffries NO, Greenstein DK, Clasen LS, Blumenthal JD, James RS, Ebens CL, Walter JM, Zijdenbos A, Evans AC, Giedd JN, Rapoport JL: Developmental trajectories of brain volume abnormalities in children and adolescents with attention-deficit/hyperactivity disorder. JAMA 2002;288:1740–1748.

9 Gogtay N, Giedd JN, Lusk L, Hayashi KM, Greenstein D, Vaituzis AC, Nugent TF 3rd, Herman DH, Clasen LS, Toga AW, Rapoport JL, Thompson PM: Dynamic mapping of human cortical development during childhood through early adulthood. Proc Natl Acad Sci USA 2004;101:8174–8179.

10 Evans AC, Brain Development Cooperative Group: The NIH MRI study of normal brain development. Neuroimage 2006;30:184–202.

11 Almli CR, Rivkin MJ, McKinstry RC, Brain Development Cooperative Group: The NIH MRI study of normal brain development (Objective-2): newborns, infants, toddlers, and preschoolers. Neuroimage 2007;35:308–325.

12 Wilke M, Krageloh-Mann I, Holland SK: Global and local development of gray and white matter volume in normal children and adolescents. Exp Brain Res 2007;178:296–307.

13 Wilke M, Holland SK, Myseros JS, Schmithorst VJ, Ball WS Jr: Functional magnetic resonance imaging in pediatrics. Neuropediatrics 2003;34:225–233.

14 MRC Ethics Guide: Medical research involving children; document available at www.mrc.ac.uk.

15 Illes J, Kirschen MP, Edwards E, Stanford LR, Bandettini P, Cho MK, Ford PJ, Glover GH, Kulynych J, Macklin R, Michael DB, Wolf SM: Incidental findings in brain imaging research. Science 2006;311:783–784.

16 Kim BS, Illes J, Kaplan RT, Reiss A, Atlas SW: Incidental findings on pediatric MR images of the brain. AJNR Am J Neuroradiol 2002;23:1674–1677.

17 Weber F, Knopf H: Incidental findings in magnetic resonance imaging of the brains of healthy young men. J Neurol Sci 2006;240: 81–84.
18 NIH guideline: Detection and disclosure of incidental findings in neuroimaging research. www.ninds.nih.gov/news_and_events/proceedings/ifexecsummary.htm.
19 Byars AW, Holland SK, Strawsburg RH, Bommer W, Dunn RS, Schmithorst VJ, Plante E: Practical aspects of conducting large-scale functional magnetic resonance imaging studies in children. J Child Neurol 2002; 17:885–890.
20 Lange N, Giedd JN, Castellanos FX, Vaituzis AC, Rapoport JL: Variability of human brain structure size: ages 4–20 years. Psychiatry Res 1997;4:1–12.
21 Wilke M, Holland SK: Variability of gray and white matter during normal development: a voxel-based MRI analysis. Neuroreport 2003;14:1887–1890.
22 Courchesne E, Plante E: Measurement and analysis issues in neurodevelopmental magnetic resonance imaging; in Thatcher RW, Lyon GR, Rumsey J, Krasnegor N (eds): Developmental Neuroimaging: Mapping the Development of Brain and Behavior, ed 1. San Diego, Academic Press, 1996, p 43.
23 Rivkin MJ: Developmental neuroimaging of children using magnetic resonance techniques. Ment Retard Dev Disabil Res Rev 2000;6:68–80.
24 Zur KB, Holland SK, Yuan W, Choo DI: Functional magnetic resonance imaging: contemporary and future use. Curr Opin Otolaryngol Head Neck Surg 2004;12:374–377.
25 Durston S, Hulshoff Pol HE, Schnack HG, Buitelaar JK, Steenhuis MP, Minderaa RB, Kahn RS, van Engeland H: Magnetic resonance imaging of boys with attention-deficit/hyperactivity disorder and their unaffected siblings. J Am Acad Child Adolesc Psychiatry 2004;43:332–340.
26 Falkai P, Honer WG, Kamer T, Dustert S, Vogeley K, Schneider-Axmann T, Dani I, Wagner M, Rietschel M, Muller DJ, Schulze TG, Gaebel W, Cordes J, Schonell H, Schild HH, Block W, Traber F, Steinmetz H, Maier W, Tepest R: Disturbed frontal gyrification within families affected with schizophrenia. J Psychiatr Res 2007;41:805–813.
27 Narr KL, Bilder RM, Luders E, Thompson PM, Woods RP, Robinson D, Szeszko PR, Dimtcheva T, Gurbani M, Toga AW: Asymmetries of cortical shape: effects of handedness, sex and schizophrenia. Neuroimage 2007;34:939–948.
28 Oldfield RC: The assessment and analysis of handedness: the Edinburgh inventory (in German). Neuropsychologia 1971;9:97–113.
29 Steingruber HJ: Measuring of laterality. Z Exp Angew Psychol 1971;18:337–357.
30 Triggs WJ, Calvanio R, Levine M, Heaton RK, Heilman KM: Predicting hand preference with performance on motor tasks. Cortex 2000;36:679–689.
31 Ruoss K, Lovblad K, Schroth G, Moessinger AC, Fusch C: Brain development (sulci and gyri) as assessed by early postnatal MR imaging in preterm and term newborn infants. Neuropediatrics 2001;32:69–74.
32 Bluml S, Friedlich P, Erberich S, Wood JC, Seri I, Nelson MD Jr: MR imaging of newborns by using an MR-compatible incubator with integrated radiofrequency coils: initial experience. Radiology 2004;231:594–601.
33 Mewes AU, Huppi PS, Als H, Rybicki FJ, Inder TE, McAnulty GB, Mulkern RV, Robertson RL, Rivkin MJ, Warfield SK: Regional brain development in serial magnetic resonance imaging of low-risk preterm infants. Pediatrics 2006;118:23–33.
34 Dehaene-Lambertz G, Dehaene S, Hertz-Pannier L: Functional neuroimaging of speech perception in infants. Science 2002; 298:2013–2015.
35 Casey BJ, Cohen JD, Jezzard P, Turner R, Noll DC, Trainor RJ, Giedd J, Kaysen D, Hertz-Pannier L, Rapoport JL: Activation of prefrontal cortex in children during a nonspatial working memory task with functional MRI. Neuroimage 1995;2:221–229.
36 Mazziotta JC, Toga AW, Evans A, Fox P, Lancaster J: A probabilistic atlas of the human brain: theory and rationale for its development. The International Consortium for Brain Mapping (ICBM). Neuroimage 1995;2: 89–101.
37 Wilke M, Schmithorst VJ, Holland SK: Assessment of spatial normalization of whole-brain magnetic resonance images in children. Hum Brain Mapp 2002;17:48–60.
38 Wilke M, Schmithorst VJ, Holland SK: Normative pediatric brain data for spatial normalization and segmentation differs from standard adult data. Magn Reson Med 2003; 50:749–757.
39 Kruggel F, Yves von Cramon D: Alignment of magnetic-resonance brain datasets with the stereotactical coordinate system. Med Image Anal 1999;3:175–185.
40 Ashburner J, Friston KJ: Nonlinear spatial normalization using basis functions. Hum Brain Mapp 1999;7:254–266.
41 Ashburner J, Friston KJ: Unified segmentation. Neuroimage 2005;26:839–851.
42 Staudt M, Schropp C, Staudt F, Obletter N, Bise K, Breit A: MRI assessment of myelination: an age standardization. Pediatr Radiol 1994;24:122–127.
43 Santosh PJ: Neuroimaging in child and adolescent psychiatric disorders. Arch Dis Child 2001;82:412–419.
44 Caviness VS Jr, Lange NT, Makris N, Herbert MR, Kennedy DN: MRI-based brain volumetrics: emergence of a developmental brain science. Brain Dev 1999;21:289–295.
45 May A, Gaser C: Magnetic resonance-based morphometry: a window into structural plasticity of the brain. Curr Opin Neurol 2006;19:407–411.
46 Kesler SR, Garrett A, Bender B, Yankowitz J, Zeng SM, Reiss AL: Amygdala and hippocampal volumes in Turner syndrome: a high-resolution MRI study of X-monosomy. Neuropsychologia 2004;42:1971–1978.
47 Giuliani NR, Calhoun VD, Pearlson GD, Francis A, Buchanan RW: Voxel-based morphometry versus region of interest: a comparison of two methods for analyzing gray matter differences in schizophrenia. Schizophr Res 2005;74:135–147.
48 Eckert MA, Leonard CM, Wilke M, Eckert M, Richards T, Richards A, Berninger V: Anatomical signatures of dyslexia in children: unique information from manual and voxel based morphometry brain measures. Cortex 2005;41:304–315.
49 Wilke M, Sohn JH, Byars AW, Holland SK: Bright spots: correlations of gray matter volume with IQ in a normal pediatric population. Neuroimage 2003;20:202–215.
50 Sowell ER, Peterson BS, Kan E, Woods RP, Yoshii J, Bansal R, Xu D, Zhu H, Thompson PM, Toga AW: Sex differences in cortical thickness mapped in 176 healthy individuals between 7 and 87 years of age. Cereb Cortex 2007;17:1550–1560.
51 Shaw P, Greenstein D, Lerch J, Clasen L, Lenroot R, Gogtay N, Evans A, Rapoport J, Giedd J: Intellectual ability and cortical development in children and adolescents. Nature 2006;440:676–679.
52 Greenstein D, Lerch J, Shaw P, Clasen L, Giedd J, Gochman P, Rapoport J, Gogtay N: Childhood onset schizophrenia: cortical brain abnormalities as young adults. J Child Psychol Psychiatry 2006;47:1003–1012.
53 Geller DA: Obsessive-compulsive and spectrum disorders in children and adolescents. Psychiatr Clin North Am 2006;29:353–370.
54 Mitterschiffthaler MT, Ettinger U, Mehta MA, Mataix-Cols D, Williams SC: Applications of functional magnetic resonance imaging in psychiatry. J Magn Reson Imaging 2006;23:851–861.
55 Neiss M, Rowe DC: Parental education and child's verbal IQ in adoptive and biological families in the National Longitudinal Study of Adolescent Health. Behav Genet 2000;30: 487–495.
56 Good CD, Johnsrude I, Ashburner J, Henson RN, Friston KJ, Frackowiak RS: Cerebral asymmetry and the effects of sex and handedness on brain structure: a voxel-based morphometric analysis of 465 normal adult human brains. Neuroimage 2001;14:685–700.
57 Gaser C: VBM toolbox for spm5, version 1.1. http://dbm.neuro.uni-jena.de/vbm/.

Neuroembryology and Aging

Neuroembryol Aging 2008;5:14–22
DOI: 10.1159/000116728

Received: January 3, 2007
Accepted: April 18, 2007
Published online: August 19, 2008

The Cerebellum in Chiari Type II Malformation

Michael S. Salman

Section of Pediatric Neurology, Children's Hospital, University of Manitoba, Winnipeg, Man., Canada

Key Words
Cerebellum · Chiari type II malformation · Neurological function · Spina bifida · Vermis

Abstract
Chiari type II malformation (CII) is a congenital deformity of the brainstem and cerebellum. In CII, the size of the posterior fossa is small and its contents are crowded. The cerebellar weight, volume, and cell content are reduced in CII. However, this reduction is not uniform and appears to involve the cerebellar hemispheres more than the vermis. The anatomical location of the vermis allows it to expand upwards, downwards, and along the ventral-dorsal axis when it is compressed in CII. This expansion seems to leave its ocular motor functions intact unlike the cerebellar hemispheres, which have no room for expansion and therefore undergo atrophy with consequent impairment of their functions.

Introduction

Chiari type II malformation (CII) is the most prevalent congenital deformity of the brainstem and cerebellum (i.e. the hindbrain). CII occurs commonly in patients with spina bifida (SB), a defect of caudal neural tube closure. SB continues to be an important and prevalent disorder despite the marginally decreasing incidence brought about by antenatal ultrasound screening and detection programs, the prophylactic pre-conception supplementation of folate to women planning to have children [1–3], and fortification of food with folic acid [4]. The birth prevalence of SB is about 0.5–1 per 1,000 [1].

In SB, there is disturbance of primary neurulation, defined as neural folding of the neural tube [5], and incomplete closure of the bony elements of the spine (lamina and spinous processes) posteriorly during the first trimester of gestation [2, 6]. In SB myelomeningocele, there is protrusion of the dura, arachnoid, and the neural tissue through the posterior defect [2, 6]. The defect can occur anywhere along the spine. Upper spinal lesions are associated with more severe brain dysmorphology, motor deficits, and behavior anomalies [7].

Hydrocephalus occurs in most children with CII [6]. Before cerebrospinal fluid (CSF) shunting procedures were developed, most infants with SB died soon after birth from the effects of hydrocephalus [6]. The usual causes of death nowadays are related to brainstem compression, acute hydrocephalus from shunt blockage, and renal failure secondary to neuropathic bladder [6, 8, 9]. Infant mortality from SB in the developed world is ~10–35% [2]. Survival to the 3rd and 4th decade has been reported [2].

Historical Perspective on Chiari Malformations

Jean Cruveilhier (1791–1874), a physician from Paris, described hindbrain malformations in patients with SB and hydrocephalus in his atlas [10, 11]. Decades later, Hans Chiari (1851–1916), an Austrian physician, pub-

KARGER

Fax +41 61 306 12 34
E-Mail karger@karger.ch
www.karger.com

1661–3406/08/0052–0014$24.50/0

Accessible online at:
www.karger.com/nba

Michael S. Salman
Section of Pediatric Neurology, AE 308, Harry Medovy House, Children's Hospital
820 Sherbrook Street
Winnipeg, MB, R3A 1R9 (Canada)
Tel. +1 204 787 2414, Fax +1 204 787 1922, E-Mail msalman@hsc.mb.ca

lished a report in 1891 introducing three grades of cerebellar changes associated with chronic hydrocephalus [11–13]. The first grade was cerebellar tonsil elongation and herniation down the spinal canal, currently known as Chiari type I malformation. The second grade was cerebellar vermis and brainstem displacement down the spinal canal, a deformity that is called Chiari type II malformation, which is the subject of this review. The third grade was cerebellar-cervical encephalocele, also known today as Chiari type III malformation. Chiari then added a fourth grade in 1896 [14], which was later described as Chiari type IV malformation; this term is not widely used now. It refers to cerebellar hypoplasia [5, 11, 15]. More recently, the term Chiari 0 malformation has been used to describe a group of children with syringohydromyelia without cerebellar tonsillar ectopia. These patients were found to have caudal displacement of the brainstem on magnetic resonance imaging (MRI) [16]. Chiari 1.5 malformation describes patients with tonsillar ectopia *and* caudal descent of the brainstem [17]. In my opinion, these hindbrain anomalies do not represent a graded severity of the same disease entity and it is therefore questionable whether this type of nomenclature is appropriate.

In his original description, Chiari acknowledged John Cleland, a Scottish physician, who in 1883 described a hydrocephalic infant with SB and distorted hindbrain [11, 12, 18, 19], which corresponds to the current description of CII. Chiari hypothesized a mechanism of deficient bone growth and insufficient skull enlargement as the cause for cerebellar herniation [12]. Julius Arnold (1835–1915) published a case report in 1894 of an infant with SB [12, 20]. He described herniation of the cerebellum into the spinal canal, but focused primarily on the spinal myelomeningocele and theories on its cause. The attachment of the name 'Arnold' to the malformation (i.e. Arnold-Chiari malformation) is therefore thought to be inappropriate because his writings were mainly about spinal dysraphism [11, 12].

Theories and Mechanisms of Chiari Type II Malformation

Several theories have been proposed to explain CII. Chiari proposed through his publications in the 1890s that occipital bone abnormalities might be responsible for these malformations [12]. The molecular genetic theory proposes a disturbance of rhombomeric segmentation and ectopic expression in the embryonic hindbrain due to genetic mutation [21]. Sarnat [22] found that ependymal vimentin was overexpressed only in areas of dysgenesis in fetuses and young infants with CII. He speculated that this could reflect a secondary upregulation due to defective expression of another gene. Other theories include: downward traction of the lower spinal cord which was postulated to pull the hindbrain down the spinal canal; downward displacement of the hindbrain by the effects of hydrocephalus; dysgenesis of the hindbrain, and neuronal overgrowth of the brain before neural tube closure [5, 19, 23]. These theories, however, are not comprehensive and only explain some of the CII features [23].

A popular theory proposes that crowding of a small posterior fossa is responsible for CII [23]. The small size of the posterior fossa in CII is caused by CSF leak through myelomeningocele. This leak limits the pressure generated from CSF buildup in the embryonic ventricular system [23, 24], thereby preventing the ventricular distension required to induce both neural and calvarial development [25]. The development of the bony elements of the posterior fossa in utero depends on increasing CSF pressure within the posterior fossa and does not parallel vermis growth [24, 26]. In other words, posterior fossa development precedes the growth of its contents [26].

The cerebellum differentiates relatively early during embryogenesis and does not reach its final configuration until several months after birth. After the neural tube is formed at 4 weeks of gestation, and specifically when the rostral pore of the neural tube closes, the hindbrain starts to form [27]. The vermis develops before the cerebellar hemispheres at the end of the 2nd month after conception. Cerebellar vermis lobules I–V develop earlier than vermis lobules VI and VII [28, 29].

The Dysmorphology of Chiari Type II Malformation

The origin of hindbrain abnormalities in CII is not primary central nervous system (CNS) malformation [30]. However, this view is not held universally [21, 22]. The cerebellar vermis lobules, flocculi, tonsils, superior, and inferior medullary veli are not aplastic and can be identified on MRI scans in children with CII [31].

The deformity of CII seems to occur as a consequence of CSF leakage, which results in a small posterior fossa. The small posterior fossa becomes crowded by hindbrain structures as they develop and expand. The hindbrain herniates through the tentorial incisura and the foramen magnum. This sequence of events has been supported by recent reports demonstrating reduction or prenatal reso-

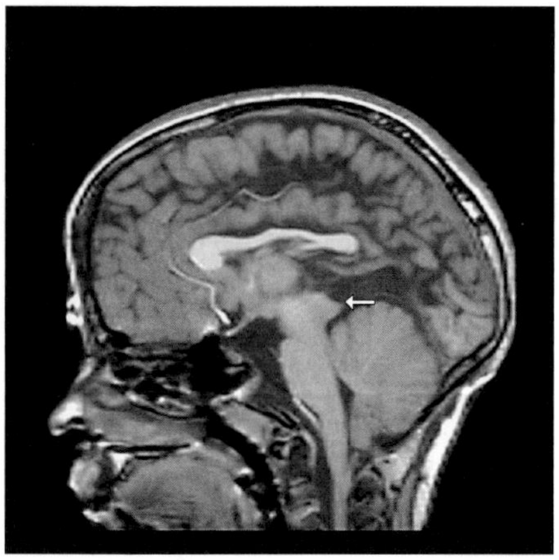

Fig. 1. Midsagittal T_1-weighted brain MRI of a child with CII illustrating tectal beaking (arrow).

lution of CII following primary repair of the spinal defect in utero [8, 32].

The small posterior fossa size in SB is detectable in fetuses as early as 16 weeks of gestation [30, 33]. CII, occurring exclusively in children with SB [6, 15, 19], can be identified early, and has been described in ~54% of fetuses with SB [30]. Ventricular dilatation may be detected in utero on ultrasound [33, 34]. It follows the development of CII and leads to hydrocephalus in 85–90% of children with CII [24]. Hydrocephalus usually presents at or soon after birth with enlarging ventricular or head size. Hindbrain herniation obstructs CSF outflow from the fourth ventricle and causes hydrocephalus [8, 33]. Hydrocephalus may also occur secondary to aqueduct stenosis or occlusion [6, 9]. Hydrocephalus exacerbates hindbrain compression [24].

The hindbrain anatomical deformity is characteristic. The brainstem is stretched inferiorly and narrowed in the anteroposterior diameter, often lying at the foramen magnum or in the cervical spinal canal. The cervical spinal cord and the medulla are displaced inferiorly forming, in some, a cervicomedullary kink [15]. The inferior part of the cerebellar vermis often herniates downward, forming a tongue of tissue posterior to the medulla that usually extends to the upper cervical vertebrae (C), at C2 or C4 level (fig. 1). The cerebellum wraps around the brainstem and is indented rostrally by the tentorium and caudally by the foramen magnum or by the posterior arch of C1 [15]. In some cases of CII, agenesis or hypoplasia of the lateral cerebellar hemispheres has been described [15].

In CII, the mesencephalic tectum (quadrigeminal plate) is often distorted, probably secondary to compression by the temporal lobes, which are expanded as a result of hydrocephalus, and the cerebellar hemispheres surrounding the brainstem. The superior part of the cerebellar vermis is shifted upwards. The tectum is stretched posteriorly and inferiorly, and appears on CT and MRI scans as a 'beak' (fig. 1) [15]. Beaking of the tectum is reported to occur in 75% of CII cases, being more prominent as the age of the affected children increases and with more extensive myelomeningocele [7, 35].

Reduced cerebellar volume, weight, and cell content in CII have been reported in many studies. The cerebellum was found to be hypoplastic in an autopsy report of a fetus at 18 weeks of gestation [30]. The volume of neural tissue in the posterior fossa in a 16-week-old fetus with SB was found to be less than one half of that of a control fetus [33]. The transverse cerebellar diameter on fetal ultrasound was smaller in 19 fetuses with SB than 17 fetuses with isolated hydrocephalus [36]. Degeneration of the whole cerebellum, also referred to as 'vanishing cerebellum', in CII has also been reported in 4 children, aged 1 month to 4.5 years, using brain MRI [37]. In 2002, Boltshauser et al. [38] reported 3 children with SB and CII, who had asymmetrical reduction in cerebellar hemispheres. One report found larger reduction in the number of cells and DNA content in the internal granular layer of the inferior vermis in comparison to the central vermis lobules in 100 children with SB, when compared with 120 controls [39]. Cerebellar weights in 100 children with SB, who died within 4 weeks of birth, were found to be smaller than the cerebellar weight of 60 control children with normal vermis who died from other causes [40]. The herniated cerebellar tissue shows Purkinje and granule cell depletion, shrinkage and gliosis of the folia, and myelin depletion [5].

One study reported smaller cerebellar volumes in 52 children with SB compared with 16 age-matched controls using volumetric analysis on MRI [41]. The study also reported that the cerebellar gray and white matter volumes were both reduced, and the reduction was greater in children with high spinal lesion levels than in children with low spinal lesion levels.

The small cerebellar size has been blamed on mechanical compression secondary to crowding. The mechanical compression is presumed to lead to secondary ischemic changes and thus parenchymal loss. Remarkably, the cerebellar loss affects the cerebellar hemisphere, and usually spares the vermis [38, 39].

Table 1. Mean (SD) values of midsagittal MRI parameters in the control and CII groups

MRI parameters	Control group	CII group	Change, %	p value
Transverse distance across the vermis	30.9 ± 5.30	36.8 ± 5.5	19.1	<0.0001
Longitudinal distance across the vermis	55.6 ± 5.8	67.0 ± 9.1	20.5	<0.0001
Herniation distance	0	17.1 ± 7.9	100	<0.0001
Intracranial area	15,397 ± 1,148	16,101 ± 1,434	4.6	0.023
Posterior fossa area	3,291 ± 308	2,993 ± 487	–9.1	0.003
Cerebellar vermis	1,391 ± 192	1,740 ± 345	25.1	<0.0001
Area of lobules I–V	473 ± 68	620 ± 148	31.1	<0.0001
Area of lobules VI and VII	291 ± 35	418 ± 106	43.6	<0.0001
Herniation area	0	164 ± 95	100	<0.0001

Measurements are in mm for distances and mm^2 for areas based on 28 control scans and 68 CII scans, except for the intracranial area (n = 67), and areas of vermis lobules I–V (n = 66), and vermis lobules VI and VII (n = 66 scans). Change (%) = (CII – control mean values) × 100/control mean value. Significance level is defined at $p < 0.01$ on Student's t test.

Other anomalies associated with CII include lacunar skull or Lückenschädel (i.e. irregularity of the inner and outer surfaces of the skull bones), enlargement of the foramen magnum, shortening of the clivus, scalloping of the petrous bone, low-lying tentorium cerebellum with large incisura, dysplasia of the tentorium, elongated cranial nerves, hypoplasia or aplasia of the cranial nerve nuclei, syringomyelia, aqueductal stenosis, absence or hypogenesis of the corpus callosum, polygyria, cortical neuronal migration defects, cerebellar dysplasia, and large massa intermedia of the thalamus [5, 9, 15, 24].

Secondary dysmorphologies also occur in CII, some related to increased intracranial pressure [7, 15]. These include secondary atrophy of the corpus callosum, compression of the diencephalon, defects in the optic pathways, and rearrangement of the cortical architecture of the midbrain. The brain as a whole may show reduction in the thickness of the cortical mantle, reduced overall brain mass and selective thinning of the posterior cortical regions [42].

Quantifying the Cerebellum Non-Invasively

Quantifying various regions of interest within the brain non-invasively has become feasible with modern neuroimaging technology. It allows structure-function correlation in health and disease. New MRI technologies have been developed for measuring distances, areas (planimetry), and volumes of specific regions of interest within the brain. Anatomical identification of different parts of the brain on MRI, specifically the cerebellum and its lobules, and their correlation with autopsy specimens, has demonstrated its reliability and good spatial resolution [43]. Volumetric brain measurement has been used mainly in research. It is not widely available in clinical practice, though studies have been published to evaluate its use for identifying subtle brain size changes, for example, in children with autism [44] or intrauterine growth retardation [45].

Planimetry (area measurements) on midsagittal brain MRI has been used to measure intracranial contents, posterior fossa, cerebellar vermis, cerebellar vermis lobules I–V, vermis lobules VI and VII, and vermis lobules VIII–X in a variety of diseases [31, 46–56].

Measuring cerebellar volumes in CII is challenging. The dysmorphology of the hindbrain renders the identification of many of the anatomical markers that are needed for the volumetric algorithm difficult. Furthermore, CII deformity is not uniform across subjects with CII. Wide variation in CII deformity has been reported on shape analyses [56]. Thus, positioning anatomical markers across different scans for the purpose of averaging them is also difficult. Volumetric brain analysis using MRI in CII has been performed in one study [41]. It showed smaller cerebellar volumes in children with CII in comparison to age-matched controls [41].

Distance measurements have been used to quantify abnormalities in Chiari malformation to predict function or prognosis. Herniation distances below the foramen magnum have been reported in Chiari type I [52, 57–59] and CII [56]. Other measurements performed in CII on a midsagittal MRI scan of the brain include: longitudinal distance across the vermis, defined as a line

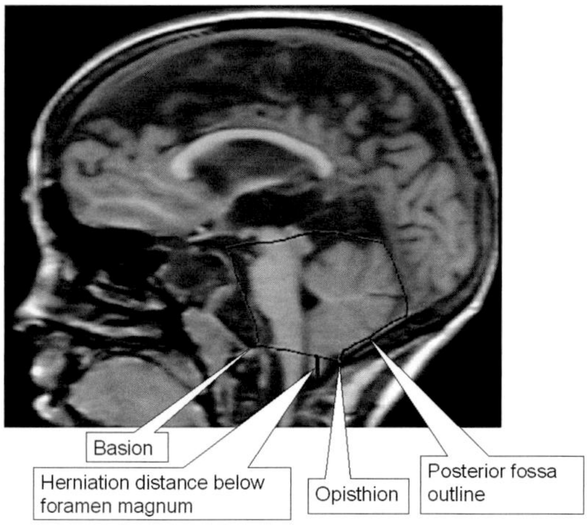

Fig. 2. Midsagittal T_1-weighted brain MRI of a child with CII illustrating the borders of the posterior fossa and herniation of the cerebellar vermis below the foramen magnum.

across the vermis joining the highest and lowest points, the length of the clivus bone, and the length of the brainstem [57, 60].

Planimetry of the posterior fossa, but not its contents, on midsagittal brain MRI has been reported in one study in 25 subjects with CII in comparison with 25 controls [56]. The mean posterior fossa area in CII was 13.4% smaller than the posterior fossa area in controls. In a more detailed study of the vermis in CII [31], planimetry on midsagittal brain MRI was performed in 68 (37 females) subjects with CII. Their mean age (SD) was 13 (3.1) years. Seventeen subjects had spinal lesions at or above T12 level and 51 subjects had spinal lesions at or below L1 level. Twenty-eight typically developing children (13 females) with a mean age (SD) of 14.1 (3.1) years constituted the control group. Measurements of the vermis and its lobules were hypothesized to be smaller in CII because many studies have shown that the cerebellum is smaller in subjects with SB, as discussed earlier. In addition, cerebellar lobules VI and VII develop last, and were therefore hypothesized to be most affected in subjects with CII. These lobules have to fit in a small posterior fossa that is already occupied by lobules I–V.

Contrary to these hypotheses, a significant increase – *not decrease* – in the cerebellar vermis area in CII was found in comparison to the vermis area in the control group on midsagittal MRI. A 25% *increase* in mean vermis area occurred *despite a smaller* posterior fossa area (table 1). This increase involved longitudinal and transverse expansion of the midsagittal vermis, and persisted after taking the area of the intracranial fossa into consideration. All midsagittal vermis lobule areas were larger in participants with CII than in controls. Therefore, the increase in the entire midsagittal vermis area cannot be blamed on inferior vermis herniation. Quantitative analyses of CII on midsagittal brain MRI confirmed that the mean posterior fossa area in CII is smaller by ~9% in comparison to controls (table 1, fig. 2). A similar finding has been confirmed in earlier reports [15, 23, 30, 33, 56].

It appears that the reported reduction in cerebellar size in CII is not uniform and seems to involve the cerebellar hemispheres, which have no place for expansion and growth within the confines of a small posterior fossa. However, the vermis may be less affected than the cerebellar hemispheres in CII, because being a midline structure means that the vermis can expand upwards comprising the so-called towering of the cerebellum on MRI, herniate downwards through the foramen magnum, and expand along the ventral-dorsal axis as seen on midsagittal MRI. In other words, midsagittal crowding is apparent in CII.

Planimetry of midsagittal MRI in CII is informative, but it does not give a global picture of the deformity in CII. Different models for vermis morphology in CII are illustrated in figure 3. A larger midsagittal cerebellar vermis area can result from hypertrophy or hyperplasia of cells in the vermis. This is unlikely, however, because many studies have reported a smaller overall cerebellar size and vermis cellular content in CII. The most likely explanation for an enlarged midsagittal cerebellar vermis area is mechanical pressure that results from a small and crowded posterior fossa. This pressure generates forces that squeeze the vermis from either side towards the midline, resulting in the apparent increase in its surface area on midsagittal MRI. The deformity of the cerebellum in CII makes accurate volumetric quantification of the vermis on MRI challenging, because the medial borders of the cerebellar hemispheres cannot be easily distinguished from the lateral borders of the vermis. Therefore, the estimated vermis volume in CII in one study [41] is not likely to be accurate because the authors assumed that the deformity of CII affects the cerebellar hemispheres and the vermis uniformly. This assumption has subsequently been proven to be inaccurate as discussed above [31]. It is not known whether the midsagittal vermis area expansion is accompanied by a significant vermis volume reduction or if the vermis volume remains unchanged in CII, i.e. the vermis shape but not its volume is affected in CII.

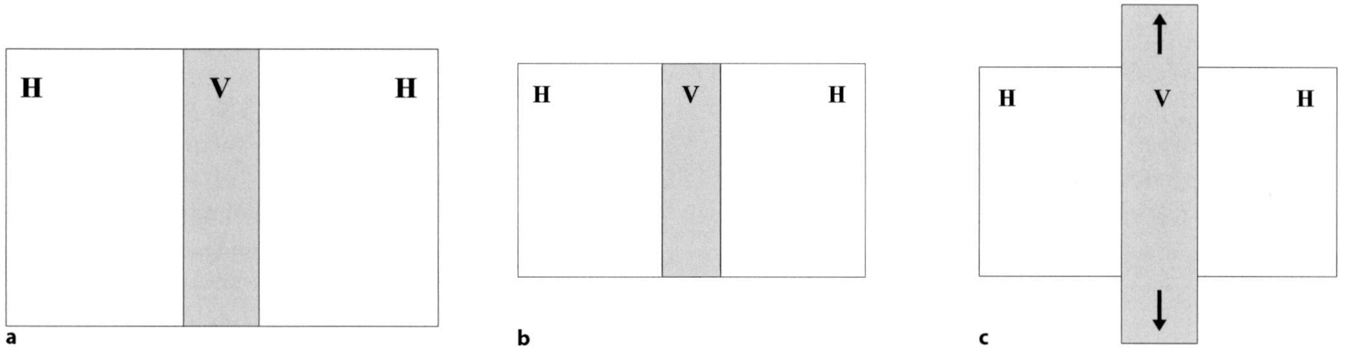

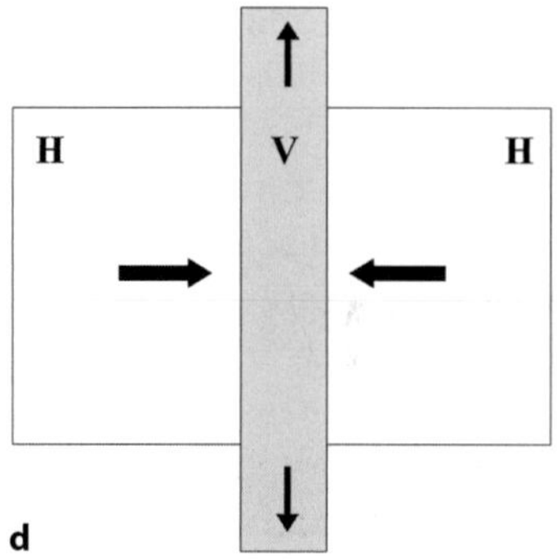

Fig. 3. Models illustrating possible morphological changes in the cerebellum in CII. Coronal sections through the cerebellar hemispheres (H) and vermis (V) are shown. The diagrams and areas are not drawn to scale. **a** Normal. **b** The widths of the vermis and cerebellar hemispheres are reduced in CII in comparison to normal (**a**). Current evidence does not support this uniform reduction in size of the vermis and cerebellar hemispheres in CII. **c** The width of the vermis is the same as that shown in a normal control (**a**), but its size is expanded. The cerebellar hemispheres are reduced in size in comparison to a normal control (**a**). The arrows depict the rostral-caudal expansion of the vermis in CII. Current evidence does not support this model because hypertrophy or hyperplasia of the vermis does not occur in CII. **d** The width of the vermis is reduced in CII in comparison to that shown in a normal control (**a**), but its midsagittal size is larger. The arrows depict the change in CII and show vermis compression (horizontal arrows) and rostral-caudal expansion (vertical arrows). Current evidence supports this model. It is not known whether the midsagittal vermis area expansion is accompanied by vermis volume reduction or if vermis volume remains unchanged in CII. (Reprinted after modification from Salman et al. [31, fig. 5, p. 391], copyright Springer-Verlag 2005, with kind permission of Springer Science and Business Media.)

These findings may have implications on cerebellar function in subjects with CII. Cerebellar functions served by the vermis, for example some types of eye movements and ocular motor learning [61, 62], may be less affected by the deformity in CII than cerebellar hemispheric functions, for example, coordination of voluntary limb movements, speech, language, and cognitive processing [61, 62], because the vermis has room to expand when it is compressed as a result of a small posterior fossa.

Are the Brain Deficits in SB Caused by Cerebellar Dysfunction? And Does the Volume Reduction in the Cerebellar Hemispheres Impair Their Function in Chiari Type II Malformation?

There is some evidence against the cerebellar malformation of CII being the *main cause* of functional deficits in subjects with SB [63]. These neurological deficits can result from widespread primary brain abnormalities that also occur in SB, for example complete or partial agenesis of the corpus callosum, syringobulbia (i.e. the fluid cavity within the brainstem), and neuronal migration defects [9, 15, 64, 65]. Furthermore, secondary dysmorphologies also occur in SB. Some of these are related to increased intracranial pressure [15, 66], for example secondary atrophy of the corpus callosum and beaking of the superior colliculus. Congenital hydrocephalus occurs in most children with CII, and has detrimental effects on the developing brain [67, 68]. The brain as a whole may show reductions in the thickness of the cerebral cortical mantle, reduced overall brain mass, and selective thinning of posterior cerebral cortical regions [15, 42]. These abnormalities might be responsible, at least in part, for the cognitive and upper limb motor abnormalities documented in SB [7, 63, 69].

On the other hand, there is evidence for cerebellar dysfunction being the cause for some fundamental brain deficits in subjects with SB. Evidence is accumulating for a cerebellar role in cognition [70–72]. In addition, the cerebellum participates in the timing of motor and cognitive processes [73–76]. Perception and motor timing deficits have both been reported in subjects with SB [41]. Indeed, the timing deficits that result from cerebellar involvement may be responsible for cognitive dysfunction in SB [41]. Further, cerebellar skeletal motor [63] and speech [77] deficits are features of CII. Case reports of eye movement abnormalities in CII, such as nystagmus and saccadic hypermetria, also implicate cerebellar dysfunction in SB [64, 65, 78].

Cerebellar volume reduction and cell loss have been documented in few studies, as discussed earlier. In an autopsy report of 25 infants with CII aged less than 2 years [9], cerebellar dysplasia was described in the form of heterotopias (displaced but well-formed cerebellar folia), heterotaxia (disordered combination of mature neurons and germinal cells), and immature germinal cell collections. However, those 25 infants were not a representative sample of children with CII since they were very severely affected and died at an early age. Furthermore, cerebellar dysplasia has been reported in 194 infants with apparently normal neurological function who died from nonneurological causes [79]. Another neuropathological study on fetuses without evidence of disease or malformation, obtained from therapeutic abortions, also reported that midline focal cerebellar dysplasias are normal variants of development [80]. It appears that cerebellar dysplasia is not a good predictor of cerebellar function.

Does the Chronic Mechanical Compression within the Posterior Fossa in Chiari Type II Malformation Impair Vermis Function?

A few reports have indicated that the vermis is only mildly affected by the deformity in CII on MRI and autopsy [38, 39]. Although the vermis is involved in coordinating gait, subjects with SB myelomeningocele have a spinal cord defect that causes upper and lower motor neuron lesions, which impair their ambulation. Therefore, the effects of the deformity in CII on gait cannot be investigated easily, accurately and independently of the spinal cord lesion.

Saccades are fast eye movements and saccadic adaptation is a form of ocular motor learning that corrects errors in saccadic amplitude [81, 82]. Mounting evidence suggests that the ocular motor vermis (vermis lobules VI and VII) and the fastigial nuclei play an important role in processing saccadic amplitude accuracy and saccadic adaptation. Saccadic amplitude accuracy, latency, and saccadic adaptation are typically normal in most children with CII, indicating that the function of the ocular motor vermis is generally intact in CII [81, 82]. These results are concordant with the MRI results of vermis expansion in CII leading to preserved function.

Therefore, the vermis may be distorted and compressed in CII, but its physiological role in processing saccadic amplitude and its adaptation remains typically unaffected. The morphological abnormalities in CII are congenital, develop slowly, and cause ocular motor vermis expansion on midsagittal MRI without impairing saccades and their adaptation. An alternative explanation of the results of these investigations is that despite the deformity in CII, reserved neural function in the cerebellum suffices for normal saccadic processing to occur. Interestingly, two recent studies on tasks that involve the cerebellum [83, 84] also reported normal motor learning of visually guided reaching, mirror drawing, and weight judgments in children with CII.

Conclusions

In sum, there is evidence for partial impairment in cerebellar function in CII. CII appears to affect cerebellar function *differentially*: Ocular motor functions of the vermis and fastigial nucleus are not typically affected by CII, while skeletal motor, speech, and cognitive functions are impaired from involvement of the cerebellar hemispheres. This is consistent with the structural changes within the cerebellum in CII.

Acknowledgments

I thank Dr. M.R. Del Bigio for editing the manuscript.

Support was provided by the Spina Bifida and Hydrocephalus Association of Canada; Bloorview MacMillan Hospital foundation grants (M.S. Salman), and NIH grant 'Spina Bifida: Cognitive and Neurobiological Variability' (J. Fletcher, M. Dennis), which supported the author indirectly by providing the infrastructure for his research.

References

1 Abramsky L, Botting B, Chapple J, Stone D: Has advice on periconceptional folate supplementation reduced neural-tube defects? Lancet 1999;354:998–999.

2 Botto LD, Moore CA, Khoury MJ, Erickson JD: Neural-tube defects. N Engl J Med 1999; 341:1509–1519.

3 Lawrence JM, Petitti DB, Watkins M, Umekubo MA: Trends in serum folate after food fortification. Lancet 1999;354:915–916.

4 Mills JL, Signore C: Neural tube defect rates before and after food fortification with folic acid. Birth Defects Res A Clin Mol Teratol 2004;70:844–845.

5 Harding BN, Copp AJ: Malformations; in Graham DI, Lantos PL (eds): Greenfield's Neuropathology. London, Arnold, 2002, pp 376–386.

6 Wagner W, Schwarz M, Perneczky A: Primary myelomeningocele closure and consequences. Curr Opin Urol 2002;12:465–468.

7 Fletcher JM, Dennis M, Northrup H, Barnes MA, Hannay HJ, Landry S, Copeland K, Blaser SE, Kramer LA, Brandt ME, Francis DJ: Spina bifida: genes, brain, and development. Int Rev Res Ment Retard 2004;29:63–117.

8 Sutton LN, Adzick NS, Bilaniuk LT, Johnson MP, Crombleholme TM, Flake AW: Improvement in hindbrain herniation demonstrated by serial fetal magnetic resonance imaging following fetal surgery for myelomeningocele. JAMA 1999;282:1826–1831.

9 Gilbert JN, Jones KL, Rorke LB, Chernoff GF, James HE: Central nervous system anomalies associated with meningomyelocele, hydrocephalus, and the Arnold-Chiari malformation: reappraisal of theories regarding the pathogenesis of posterior neural tube closure defects. Neurosurgery 1986;18: 559–564.

10 Cruveilhier LJB: L'anatomie pathologique du corps humain, description avec figures lithographiées et coloriées, diverses altérations morbides dont le corps humain et susceptible. 2 vols. Paris, Baillière, 1829–1842.

11 Pearce JMS: Arnold Chiari, or 'Cruveilhier Cleland Chiari' malformation. J Neurol Neurosurg Psychiatry 2000;68:13–16.

12 Arnett B: Arnold-Chiari malformation. Arch Neurol 2003;60:898–900.

13 Chiari H: Über Veränderungen des Kleinhirns infolge von Hydrocephalie des Grosshirns. Dtsch Med Wochenschr 1891;17: 1172–1175.

14 Chiari H: Über Veränderungen des Kleinhirns, des Pons und der Medulla oblongata infolge von congenitaler Hydrocephalie des Grosshirns. Denkschr K Akad Wiss Wien Math Naturw 1896;63:71–116.

15 Barkovich AJ: Congenital malformations of the brain and skull/congenital anomalies of the spine; in Barkovich AJ (ed): Pediatric Neuroimaging. Philadelphia, Lippincott Williams & Wilkins, 2000, pp 330–337.

16 Tubbs RS, Elton S, Grabb P, Dockery SE, Bartolucci AA, Oakes WJ: Analysis of the posterior fossa in children with the Chiari 0 malformation. Neurosurgery 2001;48: 1050–1055.

17 Tubbs RS, Iskandar BJ, Bartolucci AA, Oakes WJ: A critical analysis of the Chiari 1.5 malformation. J Neurosurg 2004;101(suppl 2): 179–183.

18 Cleland J: Contributions to the study of spina bifida, encephalocoele, and anencephalus. J Anat Physiol 1883;17:257–291.

19 Gardner E, O'Rahilly R, Prolo D: The Dandy-Walker and Arnold-Chiari malformations: clinical, developmental, and teratological considerations. Arch Neurol 1975;32: 393–407.

20 Arnold J: Myelocyste, Transposition von Gewebskeimen und Sympodie. Beitr Pathol Anat 1894;16:1–28.

21 Sarnat HB: Molecular genetic classification of central nervous system malformations. J Child Neurol 2000;15:675–687.

22 Sarnat HB: Regional ependymal upregulation of vimentin in Chiari II malformation, aqueductal stenosis, and hydromyelia. Pediatr Dev Pathol 2004;7:48–60.

23 McLone DG, Knepper PA: The cause of Chiari II malformation: a unified theory. Pediatr Neurosci 1989;15:1–12.

24 McLone DG, Dias MS: The Chiari II malformation: cause and impact. Childs Nerv Syst 2003;19:540–550.

25 Stevenson KL: Chiari type II malformation: past, present, and future. Neurosurg Focus 2004;16:E5.

26 Griffiths PD, Wilkinson ID, Variend S, Jones A, Paley MN, Whitby E: Differential growth rates of the cerebellum and posterior fossa assessed by post mortem magnetic resonance imaging of the fetus: implications for the pathogenesis of the Chiari 2 deformity. Acta Radiol 2004;45:236–242.

27 Niesen CE: Malformations of the posterior fossa: current perspectives. Semin Pediatr Neurol 2002;9:320–334.

28 Isumi H, Mizuguchi M, Takashima S: Differential development of the human cerebellar vermis: immunohistochemical and morphometrical evaluation. Brain Dev 1997;19: 254–257.

29 Lesnik PG, Ciesielski KT, Hart BL, Benzel EC, Sanders JA: Evidence for cerebellar-frontal subsystem changes in children treated with intrathecal chemotherapy for leukemia: enhanced data analysis using an effect size model. Arch Neurol 1998;55:1561–1568.

30 Hori A: Chiari anomaly type II without cerebellar herniation. Acta Neuropathol 2002; 105:193–194.

31 Salman MS, Blaser SE, Sharpe JA, Dennis M: Cerebellar vermis morphology in children with spina bifida and Chiari type II malformation. Childs Nerv Syst 2006;22:385–393.

32 Bruner JP, Tulipan N, Paschall RL, Boehm FH, Walsh WF, Silva SR, Hernanz-Schulman M, Lowe LH, Reed GW: Fetal surgery for myelomeningocele and the incidence of shunt-dependent hydrocephalus. JAMA 1999;282:1819–1825.

33 Brocklehurst G: A quantitative study of a spina bifida foetus. J Pathol 1969;99:205–211.

34 Coniglio SJ, Anderson SM, Ferguson JE: Developmental outcomes of children with myelomeningocele: prenatal predictors. Am J Obstet Gynecol 1997;177:319–326.

35 Adeloye A: Mesencephalic spur (beaking deformity of the tectum) in Arnold-Chiari malformation. J Neurosurg 1976;45:315–320.

36 Pilu G, Romero R, Reece EA, Goldstein I, Hobbins JC, Bovicelli L: Subnormal cerebellum in fetuses with spina bifida. Am J Obstet Gynecol 1988;158:1052–1056.

37 Sener RN: Cerebellar agenesis versus vanishing cerebellum in Chiari II malformation. Comput Med Imaging Graph 1995;19:491–494.

38 Boltshauser E, Schneider J, Kollias S, Waibel P, Weissert M: Vanishing cerebellum in myelomeningocele. Eur J Paediatr Neurol 2002; 6:109–113.

39 Emery JL, Gadsdon DR: A quantitative study of the cell population of the cerebellum in children with myelomeningocele. Dev Med Child Neurol 1975;15(suppl 29):20–25.

40 Variend S, Emery JL: The weight of the cerebellum in children with myelomeningocele. Dev Med Child Neurol 1973;15(suppl 29):77–83.

41 Dennis M, Edelstein K, Hetherington R, Copeland K, Frederick J, Blaser SE, Kramer LA, Drake JM, Brandt M, Fletcher JM: Neurobiology of perceptual and motor timing in children with spina bifida in relation to cerebellar volume. Brain 2004;127:1–10.

42 Fletcher JM, McCauley SR, Brandt ME, Bohan TP, Kramer LA, Francis DJ, Thorstad K, Brookshire BL: Regional brain tissue composition in children with hydrocephalus: relationships with cognitive development. Arch Neurol 1996;53:549–557.

43 Courchesne E, Press GA, Murakami J, Berthoty D, Grafe M, Wiley CA, Hesselink JR: The cerebellum in sagittal plane–anatomic-MR correlation: 1. The vermis. Am J Roentgenol 1989;153:829–835.

44 Sparks BF, Friedman SD, Shaw DW, Aylward EH, Echelard D, Artru AA, Maravilla KR, Giedd JN, Munson J, Dawson G, Dager SR: Brain structural abnormalities in young children with autism spectrum disorder. Neurology 2002;59:184–192.

45 Toft PB, Leth H, Ring PB, Peitersen B, Lou HC, Henriksen O: Volumetric analysis of the normal infant brain and in intrauterine growth retardation. Early Hum Dev 1995;43: 15–29.
46 Raz N, Torres IJ, Spencer WD, White K, Acker JD: Age-related regional differences in cerebellar vermis observed in vivo. Arch Neurol 1992;49:412–416.
47 Courchesne E, Saitoh O, Yeung-Courchesne R, Press GA, Lincoln AJ, Haas RH, Schreibman L: Abnormality of cerebellar vermian lobules VI and VII in patients with infantile autism: identification of hypoplastic and hyperplastic subgroups with MR imaging. Am J Roentgenol 1994;162:123–130.
48 Jacobsen LK, Giedd JN, Berquin PC, Krain AL, Hamburger SD, Kumra S, Rapoport JL: Quantitative morphology of the cerebellum and fourth ventricle in childhood-onset schizophrenia. Am J Psychiatry 1997;154: 1663–1669.
49 Berquin PC, Giedd JN, Jacobsen LK, Hamburger SD, Krain AL, Rapoport JL, Castellanos FX: Cerebellum in attention-deficit hyperactivity disorder: a morphometric MRI study. Neurology 1998;50:1087–1093.
50 Mostofsky SH, Mazzocco MM, Aakalu G, Warsofsky IS, Denckla MB, Reiss AL: Decreased cerebellar posterior vermis size in fragile X syndrome: correlation with neurocognitive performance. Neurology 1998;50: 121–130.
51 Mostofsky SH, Reiss AL, Lockhart P, Denckla MB: Evaluation of cerebellar size in attention-deficit hyperactivity disorder. J Child Neurol 1998;13:434–439.
52 Christophe C, Dan B: Magnetic resonance imaging cranial and cerebral dimensions: is there a relationship with Chiari I malformation? A preliminary report in children. Eur J Paediatr Neurol 1999;3:15–23.
53 Nopoulos PC, Ceilley JW, Gailis EA, Andreasen NC: An MRI study of cerebellar vermis morphology in patients with schizophrenia: evidence in support of the cognitive dysmetria concept. Biol Psychiatry 1999;46: 703–711.
54 Hardan AY, Minshew NJ, Harenski K, Keshavan MS: Posterior fossa magnetic resonance imaging in autism. J Am Acad Child Adolesc Psychiatry 2001;40:666–672.
55 Schmitt JE, Eliez S, Warsofsky IS, Bellugi U, Reiss AL: Enlarged cerebellar vermis in Williams syndrome. J Psychiatr Res 2001;35: 225–229.
56 Tsai T, Bookstein FL, Levey E, Kinsman SL: Chiari-II malformation: a biometric analysis. Eur J Pediatr Surg 2002;12(suppl 1):S12–S18.
57 Milhorat TH, Chou MW, Trinidad EM, Kula RW, Mandell M, Wolpert C, Speer MC: Chiari I malformation redefined: clinical and radiographic findings for 364 symptomatic patients. Neurosurgery 1999;44:1005–1017.
58 Wu YW, Chin CT, Chan KM, Barkovich AJ, Ferriero DM: Pediatric Chiari I malformations: do clinical and radiologic features correlate? Neurology 1999;53:1271–1276.
59 Tubbs RS, Elton S, Bartolucci AA, Grabb P, Oakes WJ: The position of the conus medullaris in children with a Chiari I malformation. Pediatr Neurosurg 2000;33:249–251.
60 Nishikawa M, Sakamoto H, Hakuba A, Nakanishi N, Inoue Y: Pathogenesis of Chiari malformation: a morphometric study of the posterior cranial fossa. J Neurosurg 1997;86: 40–47.
61 Topka H: Normal functions of the cerebellum; in Klockgether T (ed): Handbook of Ataxia Disorders. New York, Dekker, 2000, pp 53–75.
62 Manto M-U: Clinical signs of cerebellar disorders; in Manto M-U, Pandolfo M (eds): The Cerebellum and Its Disorders. Cambridge, Cambridge University Press, 2002, pp 97–120.
63 Wallace SJ: The effect of upper-limb function on mobility of children with myelomeningocele. Dev Med Child Neurol 1973; 15(suppl 29):84–91.
64 Lennerstrand G, Gallo JE: Neuro-ophthalmological evaluation of patients with myelomeningocele and Chiari malformations. Dev Med Child Neurol 1990;32:415–422.
65 Lennerstrand G, Gallo JE, Samuelsson L: Neuro-ophthalmological findings in relation to CNS lesions in patients with myelomeningocele. Dev Med Child Neurol 1990; 32:423–431.
66 Fletcher JM, Copeland K, Frederick JA, Blaser SE, Kramer LA, Northrup H, Hannay HJ, Brandt ME, Francis DJ, Villarreal G, Drake JM, Laurent JP, Townsend I, Inwood S, Boudousquie A, Dennis M: Spinal lesion level in spina bifida: a source of neural and cognitive heterogeneity. J Neurosurg 2005;102(suppl 3):268–279.
67 Fletcher JM, Dennis MF, Northrup H: Hydrocephalus; in Yeates KO, Douglas RH, Taylor HG (eds): Pediatric Neuropsychology: Research, Theory, and Practice. New York, Guilford Press, 2000, pp 25–46.
68 Barnes MA, Dennis M: Discourse after early-onset hydrocephalus: core deficits in children of average intelligence. Brain Lang 1998;61:309–934.
69 Wills KE: Neuropsychological functioning in children with spina bifida and/or hydrocephalus. J Clin Child Psychol 1993;22:247–265.
70 Schmahmann JD: The Cerebellum and Cognition. San Diego, Academic Press, 1997.
71 Schmahmann JD, Sherman JC: The cerebellar cognitive affective syndrome. Brain 1998; 121:561–579.
72 Scott RB, Stoodley CJ, Anslow P, Paul C, Stein JF, Sugden EM, Mitchell CD: Lateralized cognitive deficits in children following cerebellar lesions. Dev Med Child Neurol 2001;43:685–691.
73 Salman MS: The cerebellum: it's about time! But timing is not everything – new insights into the role of the cerebellum in timing motor and cognitive tasks. J Child Neurol 2002; 17:1–9.
74 Ivry RB, Keele SW, Diener HC: Dissociation of the lateral and medial cerebellum in movement timing and movement execution. Exp Brain Res 1988;73:167–180.
75 Mauk MD, Medina JF, Nores WL, Ohyama T: Cerebellar function: coordination, learning or timing? Curr Biol 2000;10:R522–R525.
76 Bloedel JR, Bracha V, Larson PS: Real time operations of the cerebellar cortex. Can J Neurol Sci 1993;20(suppl 3):S7–S18.
77 Huber-Okrainec J, Dennis M, Brettschneider J, Spiegler BJ: Neuromotor speech deficits in children and adults with spina bifida and hydrocephalus. Brain Lang 2002;80: 592–602.
78 Biglan AW: Ophthalmological complications of meningomyelocele: a longitudinal study. Trans Am Ophthalmol Soc 1990;88: 389–462.
79 Rorke LB, Fogelson MH, Riggs HE: Cerebellar heterotopia in infancy. Dev Med Child Neurol 1968;10:644–650.
80 Yachnis AT, Rorke LB, Trojanowski JQ: Cerebellar dysplasias in humans: development and possible relationship to glial and primitive neuroectodermal tumors of the cerebellar vermis. J Neuropathol Exp Neurol 1994; 53:61–71.
81 Salman MS, Sharpe JA, Eizenman M, Lillakas L, To T, Westall C, Steinbach MJ, Dennis M: Saccades in children with Chiari type II malformation. Neurology 2005;64:2098–2101.
82 Salman MS, Sharpe JA, Eizenman M, Lillakas L, To T, Westall C, Steinbach MJ, Dennis M: Saccadic adaptation in Chiari type II malformation. Can J Neurol Sci 2006;33: 372–378.
83 Colvin AN, Yeates KO, Enrile BG, Coury DL: Motor adaptation in children with myelomeningocele: comparison to children with ADHD and healthy siblings. J Int Neuropsychol Soc 2003;9:642–652.
84 Edelstein K, Dennis M, Copeland K, Frederick J, Francis DJ, Hetherington CR, Brandt ME, Fletcher JM: Motor learning in children with spina bifida: dissociation between performance level and acquisition rate. J Int Neuropsychol Soc 2004;10:1–11.

Neuroembryology and Aging

Neuroembryol Aging 2008;5:23–31
DOI: 10.1159/000116729

Received: May 2, 2007
Accepted: August 28, 2007
Published online: August 19, 2008

Imaging of the Developing Brain

Gregory E. Antonio Winnie C.W. Chu David K.W. Yeung Anil T. Ahuja

Department of Diagnostic Radiology and Organ Imaging, Chinese University of Hong Kong, Prince of Wales Hospital, Hong Kong, SAR, China

Key Words
Brain morphology · Developing brain · Functional MRI · Imaging · MRI · Spectroscopy · Ultrasound

Abstract
The human brain undergoes changes in morphology, volume, composition and function during brain maturation. Of the various available medical imaging investigations, ultrasound and MRI are most commonly used for assessing the developing brain. Being radiation-free and non-invasive, both imaging modalities allow in vivo serial examinations of the brain during maturation without health risks. In addition, MRI has the benefit of demonstrating certain functional aspects of the brain aside from examining morphology, further adding to the knowledge of brain development. This paper reviews the current main imaging investigations used for assessing the developing human brain, from the fetal stages to childhood.

Introduction

The main imaging modalities used for assessing brain development are ultrasound and MRI. Both modalities have the advantages of being radiation-free and non-invasive, and are therefore used for studying various aspects of brain development. This review will attempt to illustrate some of the clinical and research uses of these two modalities for the developing brain.

Ultrasound

Assessment of Sulcal-Gyral Maturation by Ultrasound
Ultrasound involves no radiation, hence is suitable for both prenatal and postnatal assessment of infant brain maturation (fig. 1). Assessment of brain maturity using imaging is a more reliable indicator of fetal maturity than other commonly used parameters in obstetric ultrasonography such as biparietal diameter, femur length and abdominal girth.

Further analysis of brain morphology is possible with advances in ultrasound hardware, which has improved resolution, and takes us beyond the measure of size for determining brain maturation. The pattern of convolutional development is found to correlate well with fetal maturity by gestational age given by menstrual dates [1].

The gyral and sulcal pattern of infant brain can be delineated by ultrasound towards the end of the second trimester. However, before 31 weeks of gestation, there is a variable lag of sulcal appearance shown by ultrasound and the actual evolution of the anatomical structure in the fetal brain [2]. This lag is related to poor reflection of sound by the shallow sulcal grooves in early gestation as well as poor reflectivity of the poorly developed early cortical lamination and ill-defined early gray-white interfaces [3]. The ultrasound assessment of the brain is much better towards later gestation due to better sound reflection by the steeply inclined furrows and more mature cortical architecture.

The chronological order of sonographic appearance of sulci can give a rough estimation of the gestational age of

KARGER

Fax +41 61 306 12 34
E-Mail karger@karger.ch
www.karger.com

1661–3406/08/0052–0023$24.50/0

Accessible online at:
www.karger.com/nba

Prof. Anil Tejbhan Ahuja
Department of Diagnostic Radiology and Organ Imaging
Chinese University of Hong Kong, Prince of Wales Hospital
Shatin, N.T., Hong Kong, SAR (China)
Tel. +852 2632 1035, Fax +852 2648 7269, E-Mail aniltahuja@cuhk.edu.hk

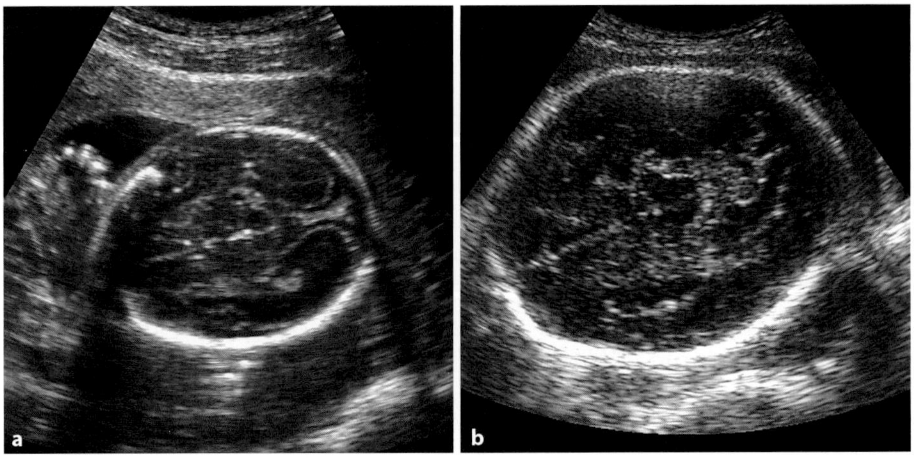

Fig. 1. Ultrasound of the fetal brain. **a** At 20 weeks of gestation, early development of lobes and ventricles is noted. Some early sulci are visible. **b** At 38 weeks of gestations, sulci and other anatomical features are completely developed.

a fetus. The sonographic complexity of each sulcus itself can also reflect the maturity of the brain. The sonographic stages of sulcal development correlate well with infant maturity as indicated by gestational age per menstrual dates. The sulcal development can be designated into three grades [4]. In the first grade, the primary sulci appear as straight lines, which are seen around 24–26 weeks of gestation. In the second grade at about 27–30 weeks of gestation, primary sulci show bending with secondary sulci branching off from the primary sulci. In the third grade at around 36 weeks of gestation, the sulci show anastomosis and branching of primary, secondary and tertiary sulci.

The most commonly identified sonographic landmark for the assessment of newborn brain maturity is the cingulate sulcus, which is easily detected on the mid-parasagittal plane (fig. 2). From 24 weeks of gestation onwards, the cingulate sulcus is faintly detected on ultrasound. It then forms better-defined, single or multiple discontinuous linear echoes. At 28 weeks of gestation, the cingulate sulcus forms a single continuous line from anterior to posterior. Its first major branch (marginal sulcus) can then be seen around this time as an upturn from the posterior aspect of the cingulate sulcus. From 32 weeks onwards, the cingulate sulcus shows arcuate configuration with multiple side branches. At term, the sulci show a complex 'anastomosed' or 'cobblestone' pattern [5]. In a study by Huang [3], 96% of the anterior cingulate sulci are seen after 25 weeks of gestation while 97% of completely visualized cingulate sulci present in infants >27 weeks of gestation; 85% of the secondary cingulate sulci are present after 31 weeks of gestation and 67% of the tertiary cingulate sulci are noted after 35 weeks of gestation.

Besides the assessment of the cingulate sulcus along the medial surface of the brain, structures on the lateral surface of the brain can also be used to assess brain maturity. Precentral, postcentral, superior temporal and inferior temporal sulci along the convexity of the brain and the progressive infolding of the opercula to close the insula and form the lateral sulcus (Sylvian fissure) are reliable indicators of surface maturity of the brain [6]. These landmarks are most useful between 24 and 34 weeks of gestations. After 34 weeks of gestation, further changes are subtle and difficult to discern.

Huang [3] has found that 89% of visualized postcentral sulci appear after 27 weeks of gestation while 93% of visualized inferior temporal sulci present after 29 weeks of gestation; 90% of the opercular closure covering the insula occur after 29 weeks of gestation, with visualization of partial and complete insular sulci after 31 and 33 weeks of gestation, respectively.

Magnetic Resonance Imaging

The most basic analysis of MRI is a qualitative analysis of the different anatomical tissue components by an experienced observer. The high-contrast resolution of conventional MRI allows good differentiation between cortical gray matter, white matter, deep gray matter and cerebrospinal fluid. With the currently available spatial resolution, small structures down to the level of hippocampal folds can be evaluated. This morphological assessment has been useful to identify normal and abnormal structures of the brain in fetal and later stages of development.

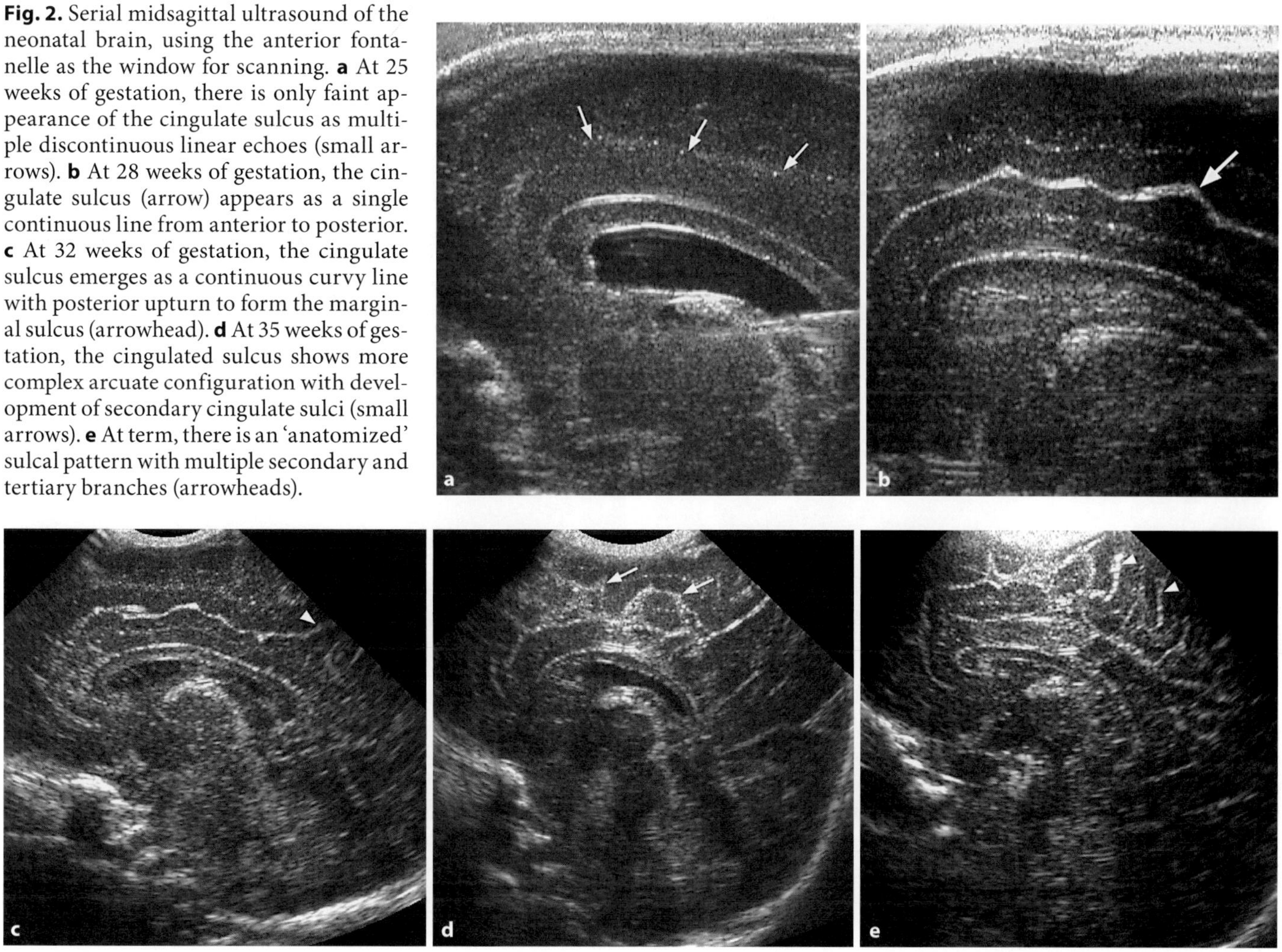

Fig. 2. Serial midsagittal ultrasound of the neonatal brain, using the anterior fontanelle as the window for scanning. **a** At 25 weeks of gestation, there is only faint appearance of the cingulate sulcus as multiple discontinuous linear echoes (small arrows). **b** At 28 weeks of gestation, the cingulate sulcus (arrow) appears as a single continuous line from anterior to posterior. **c** At 32 weeks of gestation, the cingulate sulcus emerges as a continuous curvy line with posterior upturn to form the marginal sulcus (arrowhead). **d** At 35 weeks of gestation, the cingulated sulcus shows more complex arcuate configuration with development of secondary cingulate sulci (small arrows). **e** At term, there is an 'anatomized' sulcal pattern with multiple secondary and tertiary branches (arrowheads).

Brain Morphology

MRI performed on fetuses is able to show that sulci and fissures begin to appear on the developing fetal brain around the 18th week of gestation (fig. 3). From then on, the sulci and fissures deepen and gyri become more prominent. The parieto-occipital fissure and anterior cingular fissure are the first to be visible, followed by the central sulcus approximately 6 weeks later. Secondary sulci appear around the 24th week of gestation and tertiary sulci around the 28th week. By the 35th week of gestation the primary and secondary sulci have all formed [7–9]. After birth, both sulcal and gyral patterns increase in complexity. This is believed to be due to maturation of subcortical tracts and increase in cellular density. The documentation of the normal sequence and timing of the appearance of these sulci with in utero brain MRI allows them to be used as reference for dating gestational age and brain maturation [10]. This also allows the antenatal diagnosis of cerebral hypoplasia, holoprosencephaly and cortical clefts. Aside from sulcal formation, MRI is able to resolve some of the different gray-white matter layers of the cerebral cortex during its development [11].

Brain Volume

In the beginning, brain volume was estimated manually by observers tracing the cortical outline [12]. With advances in technology, computer-aided recognition of morphometry and documentation of these tissue components are available. These programs are based on using different ranges of MR signal intensity for tissue classification. More advanced programs incorporate probabilistic atlases and surface deformation [13, 14] to improve accuracy. The brain volume rapidly increases during the first 2 postnatal years. At 3 years of age, the brain is ap-

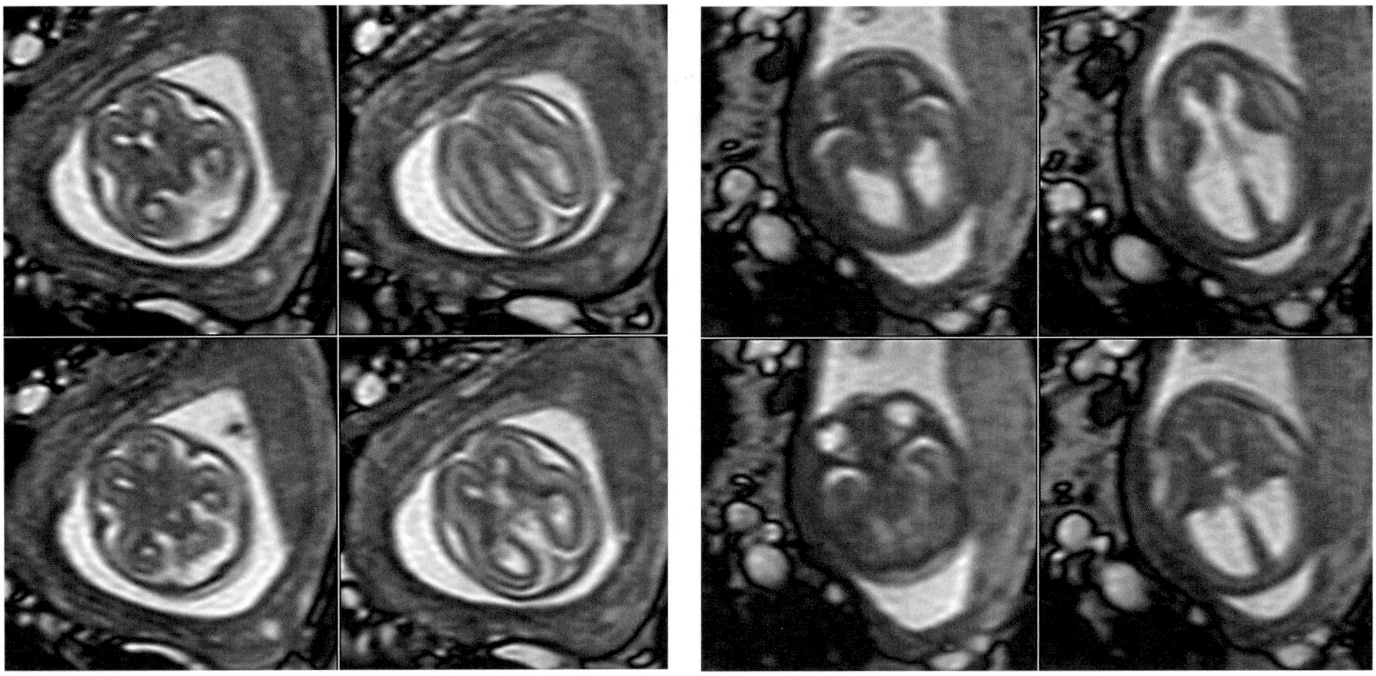

a b

Fig. 3. MRI of the fetal brain at 20 weeks of gestation with normal brain development (**a**) and at 20 weeks of gestation with dilated ventricles indicating hydrocephalus (**b**).

proximately 85–90% of its eventual adult weight [15]. Despite a relatively static weight from then on, the gray and white matter continue to remodel till the 3rd decade of life. The total brain volume reaches its peak at 11.5 years in females and 14.5 years in males [16, 17], and male brains are approximately 10% larger than females. Brain volume increases with brain maturation. Its measurement is helpful in evaluating brain developmental and degenerative disorders.

As a refinement to measuring total brain volume, the individual brain structures have been segmented three-dimensionally and their volume calculated [16–20]. The main cerebral structures of interest include: cortical and subcortical gray matter; cerebral white matter; corpus callosum, and lateral ventricles. These studies have shown that the increase in gray matter (in particular cortical gray matter) outstripped that of white matter and is the main contributor to the roughly tripling in size of total brain volume in the third trimester. The rapid increase in cortical gray matter is believed to be due to neuronal differentiation more than an increase in neuronal numbers. On the other hand, the amount of myelinated white matter increased rapidly after 36 weeks of gestation [20]. The data provided by investigations along this line have enabled more precise monitoring of brain development, aiming to better define which component is retarded or abnormal.

Brain Composition

Water Content of the Brain

Previous studies have shown that from the prenatal period to approximately 8 years of age, there is a decrease in water content and an increase in cell number [21]. MRI is highly sensitive to changes in water content and can detect this age-related dehydration [22]. More importantly, a change in the normal water content of the brain is seen in many diseases, e.g. nutritional, metabolic, infective or neoplastic ones. A good understanding of the age-related change in cerebral water content and its distribution is therefore important in helping differentiate normal development from pathology. MRI is exquisitely sensitive to changes in water content and this is routinely used in clinical practice for the detection of pathology. The age-related decrease in water content is seen as a change in signal intensity on T_1-weighted (increases) and T_2-weighted (decreases) images.

Myelination in different regions of the brain is sequential and begins in utero at the brainstem at around 29 weeks of gestation [23], starting inferiorly and posteriorly and progressing superior and anterior. For the cere-

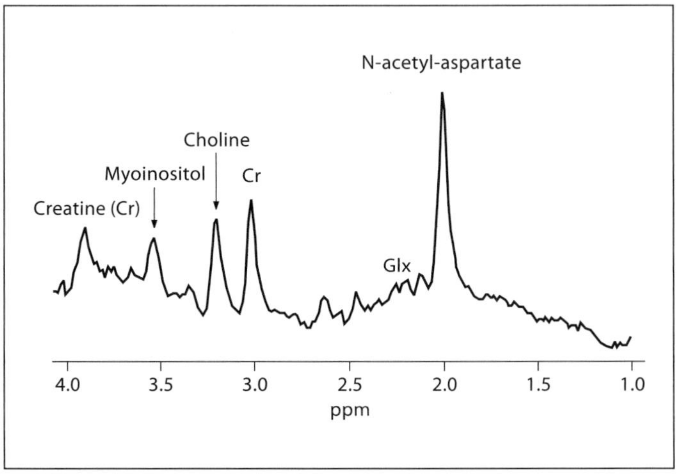

Fig. 4. MRS. This trace shows a short TE (30-ms) proton MR spectrum from the parietal lobe of the brain of a healthy 12-year-old child. The intensity of individual peaks in the spectrum is directly related to the concentration of the particular metabolite in the brain. Changes in the metabolic processes regulating the normal functioning brain may therefore be evaluated by measuring signal intensity changes of the peaks in the spectrum. Glx = Glucose.

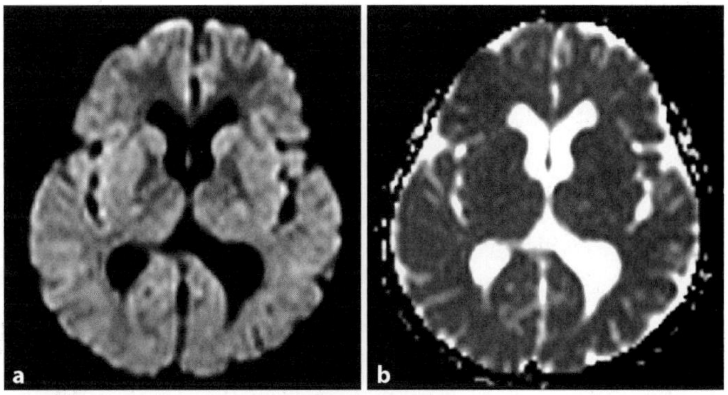

Fig. 5. a Diffusion-weighted imaging. This figure shows an isotropic diffusion-weighted image with a b-factor of 1,000 s/mm^2. Areas of the brain with the highest water mobility are depicted by regions with low signal intensity, whereas less mobile areas appear brighter on the image. **b** Diffusion-weighted imaging shown as an apparent diffusion coefficient (ADC) map. The ADC map is derived from the diffusion-weighted image in figure 4. Regions of interest may be selected on this map to obtain a direct measure of ADC values in the brain. Bright areas of the ADC map represent regions with high water diffusion as opposed to darker areas showing tissues with restricted water diffusion (a sign for pathology, e.g. edema).

brum, proximal fibers myelinate before distal ones; central cerebrum before cerebral poles; occipital before frontal poles [24–26]. Aside from regional difference, there is also sequential myelination based on function: sensory before motor fibers; projection before association pathways. Myelination occurs at its fastest pace in the first 8 months postnatally. However, axons in the cerebral cortex and certain regions (e.g. arcuate fasciculus) myelinate until the third decade of life [25].

Previous qualitative MRI studies of the developing brain have shown that gray and white matter signal intensities are reversed in the first 6 months of life when compared to the adult brain [23, 27]. That is, gray matter was of higher T_2-weighted signal compared to white matter in neonates. From 6 to 12 months, there is a sequential region-specific change to the adult pattern (white matter signals become similar to gray matter signals). The change continues until the adult pattern is reached (higher signal intensity of white matter than gray matter). These changes are believed to reflect a decrease in water content (both gray and white matter); increased myelination, and increased macromolecular precursors to myelination. Quantitative MRI studies have shown that the brain volume reached approximately 90% of the adult volume by 5 years of age. It was also shown that gray matter volume decreased and white matter volume increased [16, 17].

MR Spectroscopy

One of the major benefits of using MRI in assessing the brain is the ability to perform MR spectroscopy (MRS), which allows a non-invasive assessment of tissue biochemistry and thus infers tissue metabolism. The most widely used form of MRS uses the proton as the study target due to its abundance in the human body (in water and organic molecules). Proton nuclei, like all unpaired charged particles, have a magnetic moment. When placed in a magnetic field, protons can absorb or emit energy at a specific resonance frequency (the Larmor frequency). Proton MRS uses the principle that the same proton behaves differently in terms of its Larmor frequency when it is attached to different molecules. The different proton Larmor frequencies are therefore signatures for different molecules and can be recorded using MRS. The molecules that can be detected in this way include: choline, N-acetylaspartate, glutamine, myoinositol, lactate and glucose (fig. 4).

By recording these frequencies for a particular area of the brain, the chemical composition of that area can then be estimated. An imbalance in the chemical composition of a particular area is used for estimating the type of pathology occurring in that area. N-acetylaspartate appears to be localized in neuronal tissues and indicates the amount of intact neuronal structures. Choline is derived

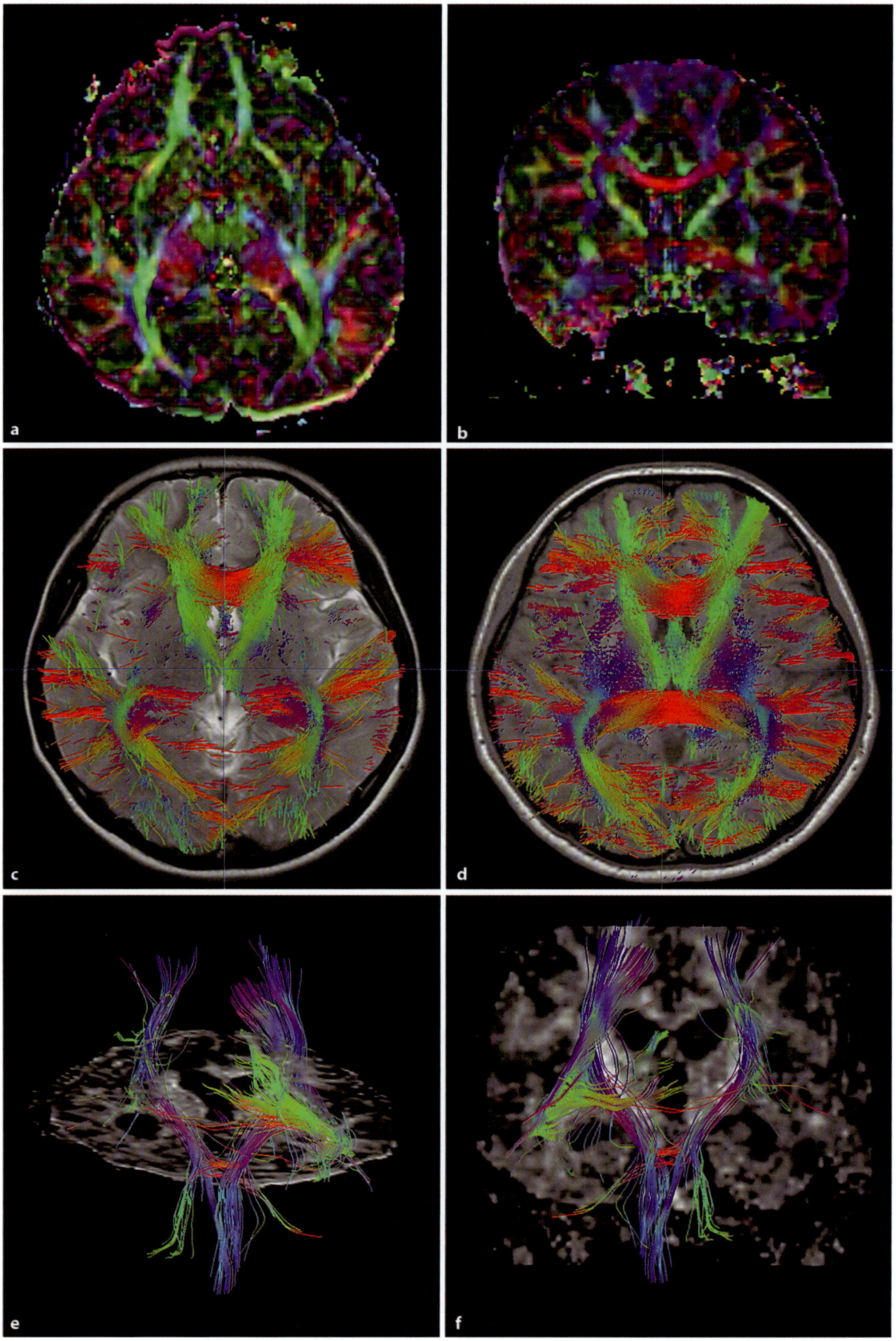

6

from glycerophosphocholine and phosphatidylcholine, components of the cell membrane. For clinical use, the relative rations of these and other molecules will suggest whether the underlying pathology is ischemia, demyelination, infection or neoplasm.

Despite these efforts to define brain composition using imaging, one should realize what is actually being measured. With the most commonly available clinical MRI units being of 1.5-tesla strength, the highest-resolution MR voxels for spectroscopy are 1 mm^3 in size. While this approaches the resolution of CT (considered the highest spatial resolution available for cross-sectional imaging), a voxel of this size in white matter would contain around 30 km of nerve fibers [28]. This same voxel in gray matter would contain around 50 million neurons [29].

Brain Physiology

Brain Water Diffusion

Diffusion-weighted imaging is a recent development in MRI and measures the three-dimensional spatial distribution of water diffusion for each MRI voxel [30–32]. The detection of water which is bound (showing restricted diffusion) indicates that edema is present within that structure (fig. 5a, b). Clinically, this is extensively used to study cerebral ischemia and infarction and their consequences in the developing brain. In terms of normal brain development, previous studies have shown that water diffusivity of both gray and white matter decreased with age [33–35]. From anatomical studies these changes reflect increases in white matter volumes for the whole brain. There is also an inverted U-shaped age-related change in gray matter volumes (increasing to a peak around 10–12 years of age and then decreases) for certain cerebral brain regions [36].

Diffusion Tensor Imaging

Despite being able to illustrate in detail the gross morphology of the developing brain (size, sulci and gyral patterns, and water content); information on the white matter fibers (such as their course or density) was not demonstrable with traditional MRI. Diffusion tensor imaging (DTI) is a relatively new technical advance, which is able to illustrate the fiber tracts of the brain using MR.

Fig. 6. Diffusion tensor imaging. These images represent fiber tracts using: color maps (**a**, **b**); two-dimensional tractography (**c**, **d**), and three-dimensional tractography (**e**, **f**). The color along the tracts (red, green or blue) represents the direction of the fiber pathways with reference to the three orthogonal anatomical planes (axial, sagittal and coronal). The signal intensity of each voxel represents the degree of anisotropy, which reflects the coherence of the fiber bundles. Signal intensity is strongest in the central regions of the tracts and weaker at the periphery.

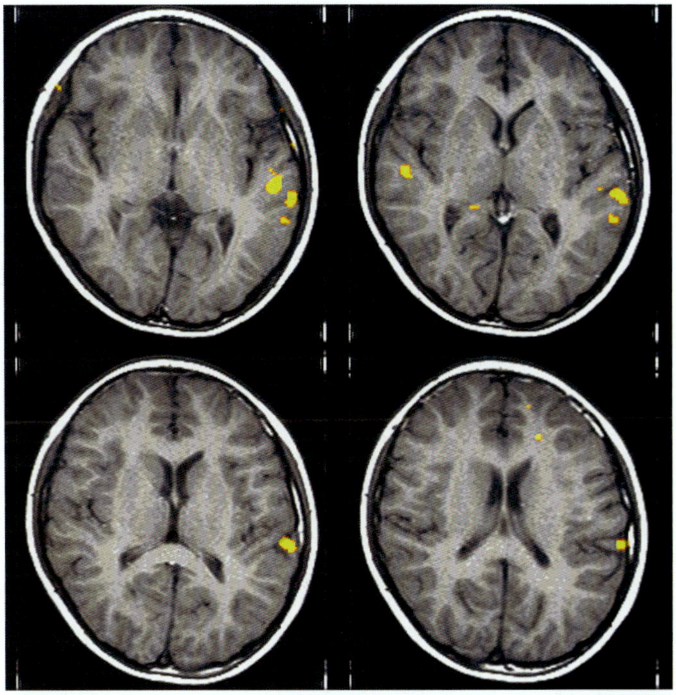

Fig. 7. These functional MR images were acquired from imaging experiments performed on an 8-year-old child while listening to English words. The active period consisted of meaningful English words suitable for preschool-age children and the rest period consisted of meaningless sounds.

DTI is based on harvesting information regarding the self-diffusing (Brownian) motion of water within axonal bundles [37, 38]. Free water such as that in the cerebral spinal fluid has equivalent diffusing motion in all directions. On the other hand, water along bundles of myelinated nerve fibers will have diffusion mainly along the longitudinal axis of the bundle (a directional restriction in diffusivity, termed anisotropy in imaging). A high degree of anisotropy (indicated by high signal) therefore indicates that the nerve bundles are paced tightly together in an orderly fashion. On the contrary, high diffusivity in the white matter would suggest poor brain development or brain pathology.

Using DTI, the diffusivity and direction of diffusion can be measured for each voxel. Mapping of this restricted water diffusion direction (anisotropy) will illustrate the direction of travel of nerve fiber bundles and thus charting their courses throughout the brain (fig. 6a, b). Tractography (fig. 6c, d) takes the mapping of fibers further by estimating the trajectories between functional cerebral regions. These tubular tracts can be reconstructed in two or three dimensions, with or without superimposition of other structures of the brain (fig. 6e, f). This ability to illustrate the different fiber tracts in the brain allows correlation between brain morphology and function, and is a particularly important advance in the study of the developing brain.

There have been many DTI-based studies performed on patients ranging from preterm infants to adolescents. For the developing brain, it appears that diffusion in white matter decreases with gestational age and with age in general [35, 38–46]. More specifically, the decrease in diffusivity was fastest in the first 2 years of life [46–48]. It is believed that this decrease in water diffusivity reflected increased myelination (associated with decreased water content), and possible axonal selection with age [49, 50], making the brain more efficient.

Functional MRI

By measuring the differences between red blood cell oxyhemoglobin and deoxyhemoglobin (the latter being paramagnetic), MRI is able to estimate regional blood flow and oxygen utilization by neuronal activity. Therefore, by performing specific tasks during scanning, specific functions can be localized to particular areas of the brain (fig. 7). This provides a true functional correlation with morphology and represents another major advance of imaging. The limitation of this imaging method is that it requires a degree of patient cooperation. This modality has found its main clinical use in the localization of functional areas close to a focal brain lesion prior to surgical resection. Follow-up studies on the reorganization of functional areas after brain surgery have also been undertaken [51]. In terms of brain development, studies on neonates have shown that the early developing brain did not show a proportionate increase in cerebral blood flow after visual stimulation when compared to adults [52, 53].

Conclusion

The advances in ultrasound and MRI have provided extensive details regarding the morphological and functional changes in the developing brain. These techniques in neuroimaging will help in our understanding of the brain and guide us in terms of treatment and protection of this vital structure.

References

1 Dorovini-Zis K, Dolman CL: Gestational development of brain. Arch Pathol Lab Med 1977;101:192–195.
2 Amiel-Tison C, Pettigrew AG: Adaptive changes in the developing brain during intrauterine stress. Brain Dev 1991;13:67–76.
3 Huang CC: Sonographic cerebral sulcal development in premature newborns. Brain Dev 1991;13:27–31.
4 Worthen NJ, Gilbertson V, Lau C: Cortical sulcal development seen on sonography: relationship to gestational parameters. J Ultrasound Med 1986;5:153–156.
5 Slagle TA, Oliphant M, Gross SJ: Cingulate sulcus development in preterm infants. Pediatr Res 1989;26:598–602.
6 Murphy NP, Rennie J, Cooke RW: Cranial ultrasound assessment of gestational age in low birthweight infants. Arch Dis Child 1989;64:569–572.
7 Levine D, Barnes PD: Cortical maturation in normal and abnormal fetuses as assessed with prenatal MR imaging. Radiology 1999; 210:751–758.
8 Garel C, Delezoide A, Elmaleh-Berges M, et al: Contribution of fetal MR imaging in the evaluation of cerebral ischemic lesions. AJNR Am J Neuroradiol 2004;25:1563–1568.
9 Fogliarini C, Chaumoitre K, Chapon F, et al: Assessment of cortical maturation with prenatal MRI. Part 1. Normal cortical maturation. Eur Radiol 2005;15:1671–1685.
10 Garel C, Chantrel E, Elmaleh M, et al: Fetal MRI: normal gestational landmarks for cerebral biometry, gyration and myelination. Childs Nerv Syst 2003;19:422–425.
11 Garel C, Brisse H, Sebag G, et al: Magnetic resonance imaging of the fetus. Pediatr Radiol 1998;28:201–211.
12 Filipek P, Kennedy D, Rademacher J, et al: MRI-based morphometry: development and applications to normal controls. Ann Neurol 1989;25:61–67.
13 Collins D, Holmes, Peters T, et al: Automatic 3-D model-based neuroanatomical segmentation. Human Brain Mapping 1995;3:190–208.
14 Davatzikos C: Spatial normalization of 3D brain images using deformable models. J Comput Assist Tomogr 1996;20:656–665.
15 Dekaban AS: Changes in brain weights during the span of human life: relation of brain weights to body heights and body weights. Ann Neurol 1978;4:345–356.
16 Giedd JN, Blumenthal J, Jeffries NO, et al: Brain development during childhood and adolescence: a longitudinal MRI study. Nat Neurosci 1999;2:861–863.
17 Giedd JN, Snell JW, Lange N, et al: Quantitative magnetic resonance imaging of human brain development: ages 4–18. Cereb Cortex 1996;6:551–560.
18 Pfefferbaum A, Mathalon D, Sullivan E, et al: A quantitative magnetic resonance imaging study of changes in brain morphology from infancy to late adulthood. Arch Neurol 1994; 51:874–887.
19 Matsumae M, Kikinis R, Morocz IA: Age-related changes in intracranial compartment volumes in normal adults assessed by magnetic resonance imaging. J Neurosurg 1996; 84:982–991.
20 Huppi P, Warfield S, Kikinis R, et al: Quantitative magnetic resonance imaging of brain development in premature and mature newborns. Ann Neurol 1998;43:224–235.

21 Dobbing J, Sands J: Quantitative growth and development of human brain. Arch Dis Child 1973;48:757–767.
22 Barkovich AJ, Kjos BO, Jackson DE Jr, et al: Normal brain maturation of the neonatal and infant brain: MR imaging at 1.5 T. Radiology 1988;166:173–180.
23 Inder TE, Huppi PS: In vivo studies of brain development by magnetic resonance techniques. Ment Retard Dev Disabil Res Rev 2000;6:59–67.
24 Volpe JJ: Overview: normal and abnormal human brain development. Ment Retard Dev Disabil Res Rev 2000;6:1–5.
25 Yakovlev PI, Lecours AR: The myelogenetic cycles of regional maturation of the brain; in Minkowski A (ed): Regional Development of the Brain in Early Life. Oxford, Blackwell Scientific Publications, 1967, pp 3–65.
26 Gilles FH, Shankle W, Dooling EC: Myelinated tracts: growth patterns; in Gilles FH, Leviton A, Dooling EC (eds): The Developing Human Brain: Growth and Epidemiological Neuropathology. Boston, Wright, 1983, pp 117–183.
27 Paus T, Collins DL, Evans AC, et al: Maturation of white matter in the human brain: a review of magnetic resonance studies. Brain Res Bull 2001;54:255–266.
28 Marner L, Nyengaard JR, Tang Y, et al: Marked loss of myelinated fibers in the human brain with age. J Comp Neurol 2003; 462:144–152.
29 Pakkenberg B, Gundersen H: Neocortical neuron number in humans; effect of sex and age. J Comp Neurol 1997;384:312–320.
30 Basser PJ, Pierpaoli C: Microstructural and physiological features of tissues elucidated by quantitative-diffusion-tensor MRI. J Magn Reson B 1996;111:209–219.
31 Conturo TE, McKinstry RC, Akbudak E, et al: Encoding of anisotropic diffusion with tetrahedral gradients: a general mathematical diffusion formalism and experimental results. Magn Reson Med 1996;35:399–412.
32 Pierpaoli C, Jezzard P, Basser PJ, et al: Diffusion tensor MR imaging of the human brain. Radiology 1996;201:637–648.
33 Huppi PS, Maier SE, Peled S, et al: Microstructural development of human newborn cerebral white matter assessed in vivo by diffusion tensor magnetic resonance imaging. Pediatr Res 1998;44:584–590.
34 Neil JJ, Shiran SI, McKinstry RC, et al: Normal brain in human newborns: apparent diffusion coefficient and diffusion anisotropy measured by using diffusion tensor MR imaging. Radiology 1998;209:57–66.
35 Mukherjee P, Miller JH, Shimony JS, et al: Normal brain maturation during childhood: developmental trends characterized with diffusion-tensor MR imaging. Radiology 2001;221:349–358.
36 Lenroot RK, Giedd JN: Brain development in children and adolescents: insights from anatomical magnetic resonance imaging. Neurosci Biobehav Rev 2006;30:718–729.
37 Taylor WD, Hsu E, Krishnan KRR, et al: Diffusion tensor imaging: background, potential, and utility in psychiatric research. Biol Psychiatry 2004;55:201–207.
38 Nomura Y, Sakuma H, Takeda K, et al: Diffusional anisotropy of the human brain assessed with diffusion-weighted MR: relation with normal brain development and aging. AJNR Am J Neuroradiol 1994;15:231–238.
39 Counsell SJ, Allsop JM, Harrison MC, et al: Diffusion-weighted imaging of the brain in preterm infants with focal and diffuse white matter abnormality. Pediatrics 2003;112:1–7.
40 Huppi PS, Murphy B, Maier SE, et al: Microstructural brain development after perinatal cerebral white matter injury assessed by diffusion tensor magnetic resonance imaging. Pediatrics 2001;107:455–460.
41 Sakuma H, Nomura Y, Takeda K, et al: Adult and neonatal human brain: diffusional anisotropy and myelination with diffusion-weighted MR imaging. Radiology 1991;180: 229–233.
42 Barnea-Goraly N, Menon V, Eckert M, et al: White matter development during childhood and adolescence: a cross-sectional diffusion tensor imaging study. Cereb Cortex 2005;15:1848–1854.
43 Ben Bashat D, Ben Sira L, Graif M, et al: Normal white matter development from infancy to adulthood: comparing diffusion tensory and high b value diffusion weighted MR images. J Magn Reson Imaging 2005;21:503–511.
44 Schmithorst VJ, Wilke M, Dardzinski BJ, et al: Correlation of white matter diffusivity and anisotropy with age during childhood and adolescence: a cross-sectional diffusion-tensor MR imaging study. Radiology 2002; 222:212–218.
45 Snook L, Paulson LA, Roy D, et al: Diffusion tensor imaging neurodevelopment in children and young adults. Neuroimage 2005; 26:1164–1173.
46 Zhang L, Thomas KM, Davidson MC, et al: MR quantitation of volume and diffusion changes in the developing brain. AJNR Am J Neuroradiol 2005;26:45–49.
47 Schneider JFL, Il'yasov KA, Hennig J, et al: Fast quantitative diffusion-tensor imaging of cerebral white matter from the neonatal period to adolescence. Neuroradiology 2004; 46:258–266.
48 Hermoye L, Saint-Martin C, Cosnard G, et al: Pediatric diffusion tensor imaging: normal database and observation of the white matter maturation in early childhood. Neuroimage 2006;29:493–504.
49 Mukherjee P, Miller JH, Shimony JS, et al: Diffusion-tensor MR imaging of gray and white matter development during normal human brain maturation. AJNR Am J Neuroradiol 2002;23:1445–1456.
50 Suzuki Y, Matsuzawa H, Keww IL, et al: Absolute eigenvalue diffusion tensor analysis for human brain maturation. NMR Biomed 2003;16:257–260.
51 Chu D, Huttenlocher P, Levin D, et al: Reorganization of the hand somatosensory cortex following perinatal unilateral brain injury. Neuropediatrics 2000;31:63–69.
52 Martin E, Joeri P, Loennecker T, et al: Visual processing in infants and children studied using functional MRI. Pediatr Res 1999;46: 135–140.
53 Born P, Miranda M, Rostrup E, et al: Functional magnetic imaging of the normal and abnormal visual system in early life. Neuropediatrics 2000;31:24–32.

Neuroembryology and Aging

Neuroembryol Aging 2008;5:32–38
DOI: 10.1159/000116730

Received: June 20, 2007
Accepted: August 8, 2007
Published online: August 19, 2008

Imaging of the Developing Central Nervous System in the Fetus

Jie Xu[a] W.H. Kwong[d] Maria Sen Mun Wai[d] E. Lucy Forster[d] Yan-ling Jiang[b, c] Hsiang-fu Kung[e] David T. Yew[d]

[a]Department of Anatomy, Zhongshan School of Medicine, Sun Yat Sen University, Guangzhou, and [b]Department of Radiology and [c]Brain Research Laboratory, Engineering Research Center of Biomedical Sciences, Kunming University of Medical Sciences, Kunming, China; [d]Department of Anatomy and [e]Stanley Ho Center for Emerging Infectious Diseases, School of Public Health, Chinese University of Hong Kong, Hong Kong, SAR, China

Key Words

Brain development · CNS · Human nervous system · Living fetus · MRI · Pregnant women

Abstract

The development of the brain was studied by MRI in living fetuses of pregnant women (performed because of medical reasons or in volunteers). They were from 21 to 37 weeks of gestation. At 21 weeks, diencephalic condensations were evident. By 25 weeks, high-density areas appeared in the prefrontal, central parietal and temporal cortices. The lentiform nucleus began to separate from the diencephalic mass between 26 and 28 weeks. The caudate nucleus, corpus callosum and septal areas were observed by 28 weeks, where the hippocampus was definitively identified by 29 weeks. By 30 weeks, the fornix was evident. Profuse CSF circulation with genesis of new gyri was noted at that stage. By 37 weeks, the brain of the fetus was much the same as that of the child except the insula did not show significant gyri.

Introduction

The detailed development of the nervous system has been an important subject on the agenda of the functional maturation of the human and, more prominently, the understanding of the mechanisms leading to malformations in the central nervous system (CNS). In spite of the many classical studies on cortical genesis, studies on regional changes in the developing human nervous system remain limited [1–7]. With the advances of magnetic resonance imaging (MRI), one is now able to gain insight into the development of the human nervous system in greater macroscopic detail. For example, Takanashi and Barkovich [8] reported that T_2-weighted images could yield details on myelination. Functional MRI has been employed in postnatal animal studies already by our group [9, 10]. D'Incerti [11], Colombo et al. [12], Righini et al. [13] and Ghai et al. [14] used MRI to study lissencephaly, polymicrogyria, agyria, pachygyria, heterotopia and hemimegalencephaly. Sbarbati et al. [15] concluded that the anatomical images obtained by MRI were useful for the study of the developing brain. The increase in the resolution of the MRI could even differentiate the genesis

KARGER

Fax +41 61 306 12 34
E-Mail karger@karger.ch
www.karger.com

1661–3406/08/0052–0032$24.50/0

Accessible online at:
www.karger.com/nba

David T. Yew
Department of Anatomy
Chinese University of Hong Kong
Shatin, N.T., Hong Kong, SAR (China)
Tel. +852 2609 6899, Fax +852 2603 5031, E-Mail david-yew@cuhk.edu.hk

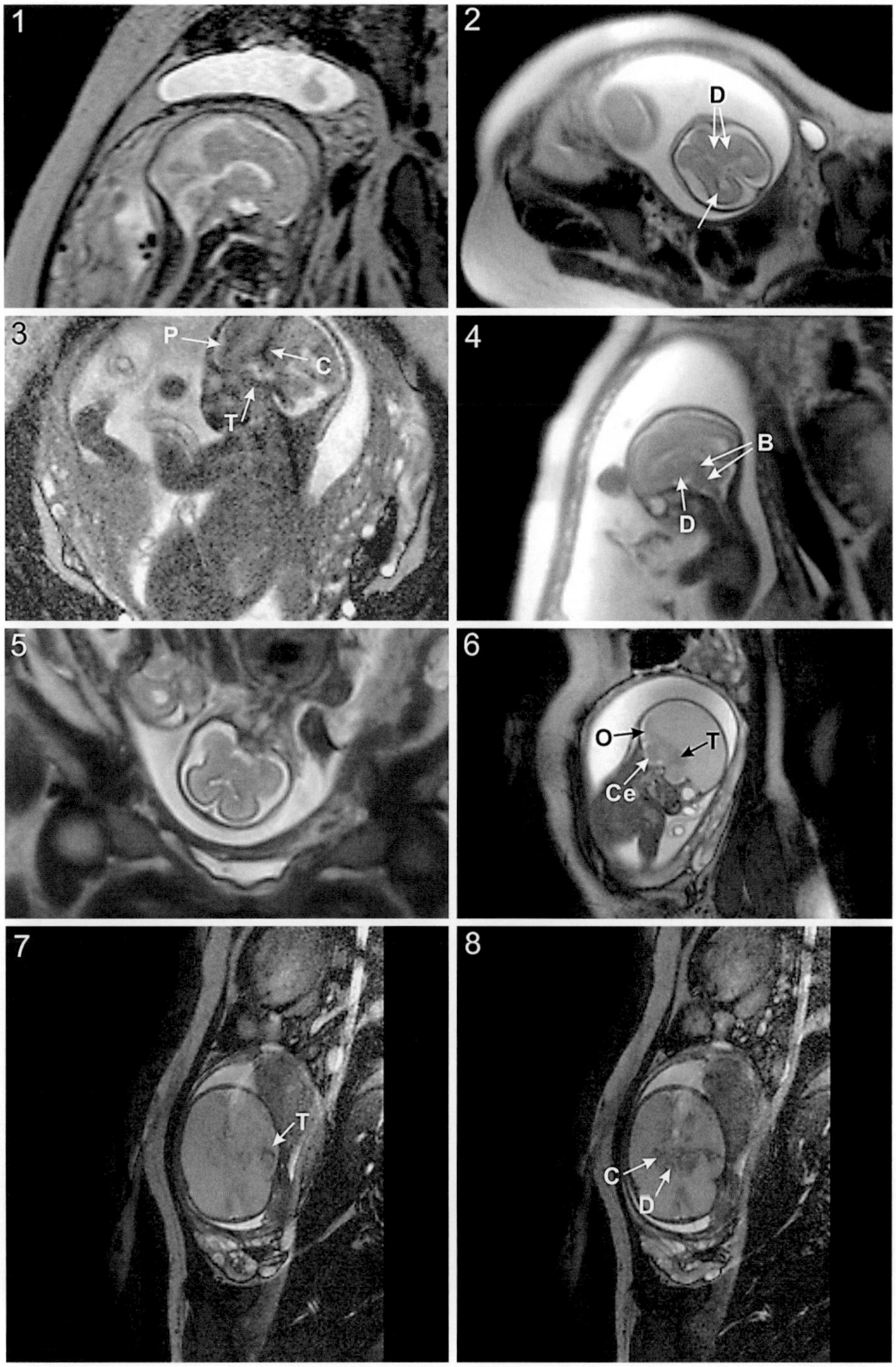

Fig. 1, 2. MRIs of the brain at 21 weeks of gestation. **1** All areas were present (sagittal section). **2** Note high-density areas in the diencephalon (D) and the medial cortex (non-labelled arrow). Coronal section.
Fig. 3–5. MRIs of the brain at 25 weeks of gestation. **3** Note high-density spots in the prefrontal area (P), around the central sulcus (C) and at the tip of the temporal lobe (T). Lateral view. **4** Some increase in density in the diencephalon (D) and brainstem (B). Parasagittal section. **5** No distinction between diencephalon and corpus striatum was visible (coronal section).
Fig. 6–8. MRIs of the brain at 26 weeks of gestation. **6** High-density areas in the posterior portion of the temporal lobe (T), occipital lobe (O) and the cerebellum (Ce). Parasagittal section. **7** High-density area was visible in the temporal area (T). Horizontal section at the base of the brain. **8** Some distinction between the medial diencephalon (D) and the lateral lentiform nucleus (C) was discernable. Horizontal section at a level higher than that of **7**.

of abnormal tracts in the defective corpus callosum [16] and reveal the differentiated regional growth rates of the cortices [17]. The schematic differentiation of the developing brain on a chronological basis as revealed by MRI was however still absent. The following paper is hopefully one of the early pieces of work on this topic.

Materials and Methods

With the consent of the mothers and the ethical committees of the hospitals, fetuses aged from 21 to 37 weeks of gestation of 30 pregnant women were studied. Fetuses aged below 21 weeks of gestation were not utilized for ethical reasons. The mothers were chosen either for medical reasons or as volunteers. The fetuses

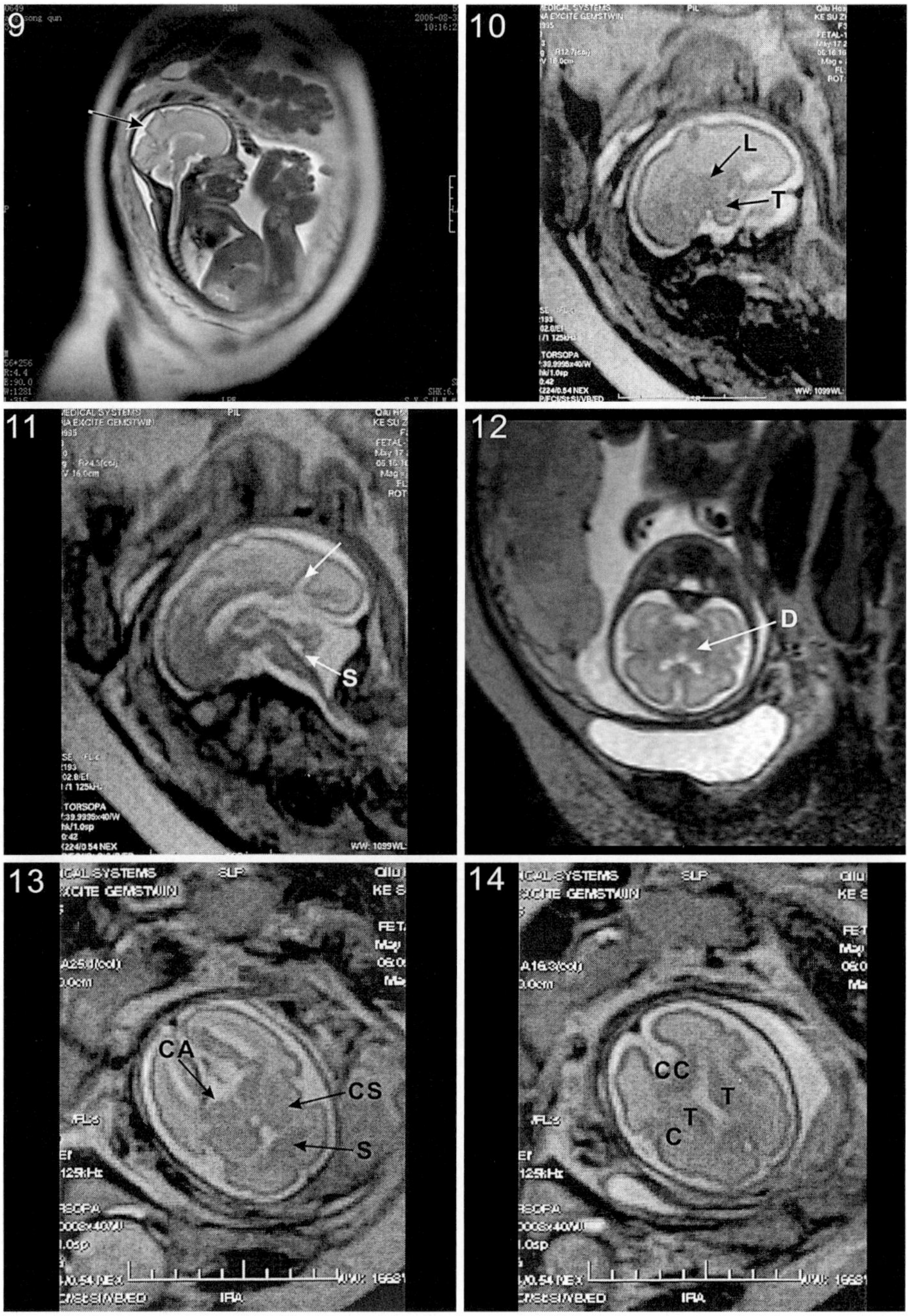

Fig. 9–14. MRIs of the brain at 28 weeks of gestation. **9** Evidence of a new gyrus (arrow). Midsagittal section. **10** High-density lentiform nucleus (L) and also high-density area in the temporal lobe (T). Parasagittal section. **11** The parieto-occipital sulcus (arrow) and the opening in the subarachnoid space (S) in the posterior medullary velum (sagittal section). **12** Diencephalic high-density condensation (D). Coronal section. **13** High-density area in the corpus striatum (CS), specifically the lentiform nucleus, the septal area (S) and the caudate nucleus (CA). Horizontal section at the base of the brain. **14** Formation of the corpus callosum (CC; splenium in this section) and the thalamic (T) and the lentiform nucleus (C). Horizontal section at the midlevel of the brain.

investigated and recorded here were all normal. MR imaging was performed in the affiliated hospitals of the Medical Faculty of the Sun Yat Sen University, Guangzhou, Guangdong Province, China.

MR imaging was performed using a Signa Excite 1.5-tesla scanner (General Electric Medical System, Milwaukee, Wisc., USA) with shielded magnetic field gradients of up to 77 mT/ms and a four-channel body coin (TORSOPA). When scanned, all the mothers held their breath. The following parameters were set (slice thickness = 5 mm, gap = 1 mm, field of view = 35 × 35). MRI images were taken using a T_2-weighted single-shot fast spin-echo sequence (TR/TE = 800/80 ms, matrix = 384 × 224, bandwidth 62.5 kHz, holding breath time = 10–20 s) and T_1-weighted fast-spoiled gradient-echo sequence (TR/TE = 200/1.6 ms, flip angle = 80°, bandwidth 41.67 kHz, matrix = 512 × 192, acquisition time = 19 s). All the mothers were in the supine position and MRI started from the lower limb up.

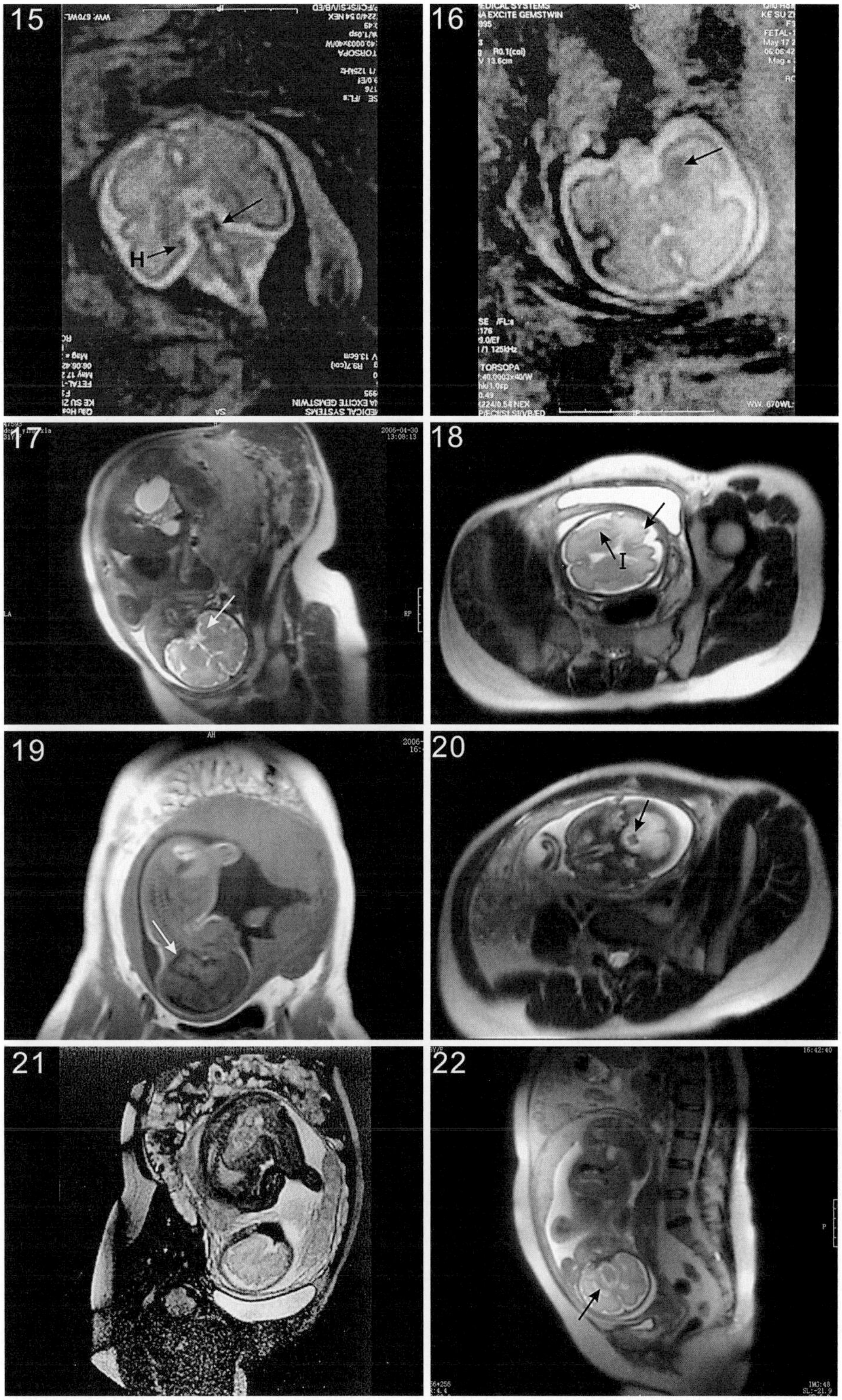

Fig. 15. MRI of the brain at 28 weeks of gestation showing colliculi (arrow) and the developing hippocampus (H). Coronal section.

Fig. 16, 17. MRIs of the brain at 29 weeks of gestation showing a definitive amygdaloid nucleus (arrow in **16**) and a growing hippocampus (arrow in **17**). Coronal sections.

Fig. 18–22. MRIs of the brain at 30 weeks of gestation. **18** Ruffling and genesis of the precentral cortex (arrow). I = Internal capsule. Horizontal section. **19, 20** CSF in sinuses leading from ventricle (arrow in **19**; horizontal section) and aqueduct (arrow in **20**; coronal section). T_2 images. **21** New gyri all over the cortex (parasagittal section). **22** Fornix (arrow). Coronal section.

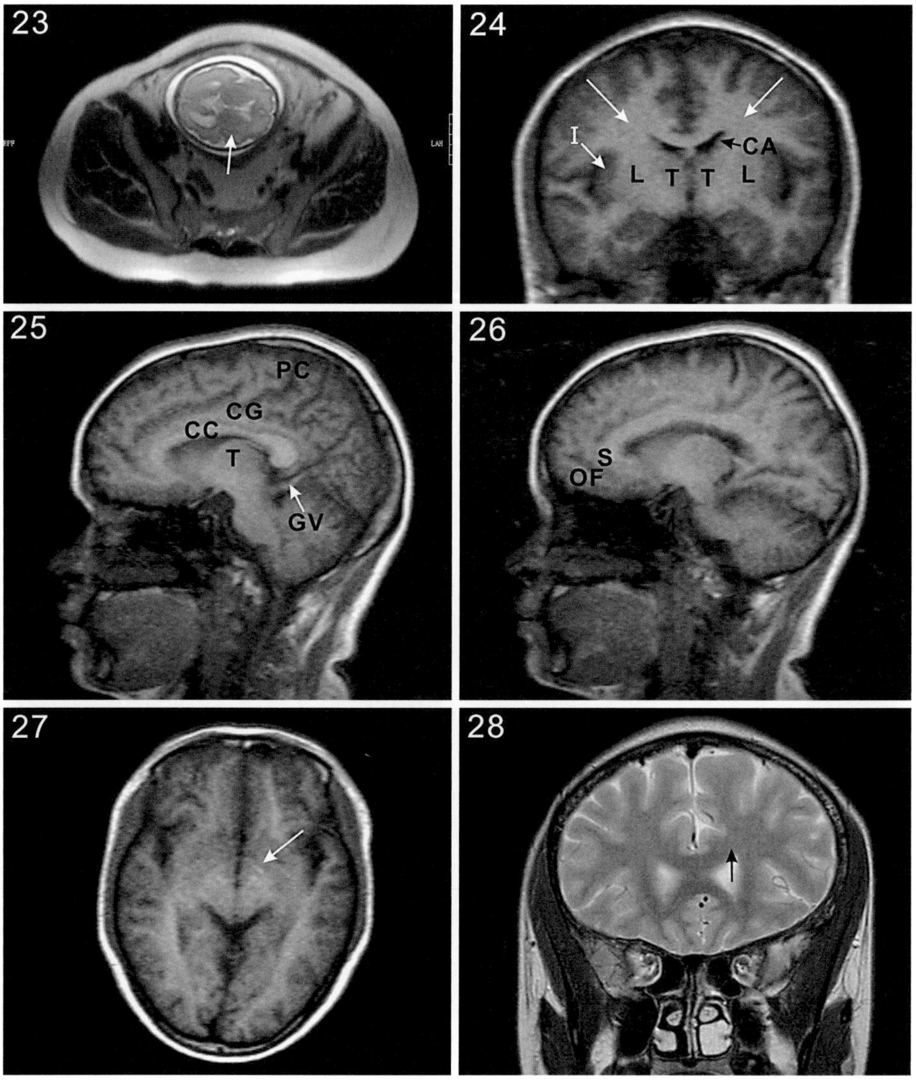

Fig. 23. MRI of the brain at 30 weeks of gestation showing an elongated lentiform nucleus (arrow; horizontal section).
Fig. 24–28. MRIs of the brain at 37 weeks of gestation. **24** Note many white fibers (arrows). CA = Caudate nucleus; I = insula without division into gyri; L = lentiform nucleus; T = thalamus (coronal section). **25, 26** Sagittal sections. CC = Corpus callosum; CG = cingulate gyrus; GV = great vein of Galen; OF = orbitofrontal gyrus; PC = paracentral suculus; S = septal area; T = thalamus. **27, 28** Arrows indicate the anterior commissure with fibers (**27**, horizontal section) and fibers in T_2-weighted image (**28**, coronal section).

Results

By 21 weeks, all major regions of the central nervous system (cortex with lobes, diencephalon, midbrain, pous, medulla and cerebellum) were observed by MRI, including the cortex and brainstem (fig. 1). Both coronal and horizontal sections revealed some high-density areas in and around the diencephalon, in the ventricular zone and in the medial cortex but not laterally (fig. 1, 2). No corpus callosum was observed. By 25 weeks, condensation of high-density spots appeared initially in the lateral cortex – prefrontal, parietal and around the central sulcus, anterior temporal lobe as well as medially in the diencephalon and brainstem (fig. 3, 4). There was, however, no differentiation between the diencephalon and the corpus striatum (fig. 5). By 26 weeks of gestation, high-density areas became very evident on the basal and posterior parts of the brains, including the cerebellum, and occipital and posterior temporal cortices (fig. 6). Horizontal sections revealed high-density areas at the base and the tip of the temporal lobe (fig. 7), the diencephalon and corpus striatum (fig. 8). By 28 weeks of gestation, the surface of the parietal area showed some ruffles, and the beginning of new gyri and sulci in the middle/posterior cortex (fig. 9). In the parasagittal section, the lentiform nucleus began to take shape (fig. 10). The parieto-occipital sulcus was very clear (fig. 11) and the medulla oblongata opened posteriorly into the subarachnoid space

Table 1. Major events of brain development evidenced by MRI

Weeks of gestation	Major events
21	Major subdivisions of the central nervous system clearly established
25	Hemispheres showed no corpus callosum High-density centers appeared in the anterior cortex, diencephalon and corpus striatum
26	High-density centers appeared in the posterior cortex and temporal lobe
28	More gyri and sulci developed Initial formation of the corpus striatum and hippocampus
29	Discrete amygdala observed
30	The internal capsule was clearly visible Distinct lentiform nucleus Heavy infiltration of fibers
37	MRI image similar to a child

(fig. 11). There were high-density spots in the future corpus striatum, including the caudate nucleus, the diencephalon, the septal area and the beginning of the hippocampus (fig. 12–15). The colliculi were clearly visible (fig. 15). Aggregation of cells into a round amygdala nucleus (fig. 16) as well as the presence of a hippocampus (fig. 17) were both demonstrated by 29 weeks of gestation. Aggregation of high-density spots was also documented in the colliculi and the medulla oblongata of the brainstem (fig. 15). At 30 weeks of gestation, ruffling of the anterior part of the hemisphere was noted and a clear internal capsule was observed (fig. 18). Profuse CSF drainage in the aqueduct and ventricles into the subarachnoid space was registered in T_2-weighted images by 30 weeks of gestation (fig. 19, 20). New gyri were found all over the cortex at this time (fig. 21). A distinct fornix began to appear in approximately 60% of the specimens (fig. 22). An elongated lentiform nucleus now emerged, clearly separated from the diencephalon (fig. 23). Heavy infiltration of white fibers was noted (fig. 24). By 37 weeks of gestation, however, the insula was still devoid of distinct folds (fig. 24). The brain at this stage was that of a newborn, with a clear fornix, corpus striatum, white matter of the cortex filled with fibers and the commissures being very prominent (fig. 25–28). The events are summarized in table 1.

Discussion

In the fetuses of Chinese origin, the average crown-rump lengths were 75–93 mm for 4 months of gestation, 100 mm for 4.5 months of gestation, around 200 mm for 7 months of gestation, 300 mm for 9 months of gestation and 350–400 mm at birth. In the present study, however, gestational ages were used as determined by the obstetricians. Crown-rump lengths for age determination were not acceptable in studies as they varied considerably in different specimens of the same gestational age. The crown-rump lengths were described here to provide a reference for readers for comparisons. From this study, although it was claimed that the presumptive components of the amygdala, hippocampus and the thalamus were recognized as early as stage 15 in human development [6] or 7–8 weeks of gestation [7], the detailed morphogenesis of such structures actually came into MRI-observable patterns much later in the life of the fetus. To the experienced investigator, histology may provide more cytological details than an MRI image. However, to typify certain cells as the precursors of a structure based on keenly observed histology alone is likely insufficient. Histochemistry or immunocytochemistry, where appropriate, should be performed. Furthermore, histological changes may result from postmortem variations as previous works were confined to fetal autopsy samples. This study dealt with living fetuses. From another point of view, MRI confirmation is a useful clinical tool for evaluating the development of the brain in the fetus.

Earlier studies by Hochstetter [1] and Hines [2] also reported early formation of the thalamus. Indeed, in this study, the earliest brain in our collection of the 21-week fetus showed high-density condensation in the thalamic region. However, unlike those reported by Hochstetter [1], there was no separation of the lentiform nucleus at 4 months. Rather, the separation was later, similar to the results reported by Hamilton et al. [4]. Using the MRI technique, we have observed condensations in the diencephalon and the surrounding areas as early as 21 weeks of gestation, but there was no distinct boundary between diencephalic regions and the lentiform nucleus. There was a continuous increase in the differentiation until around 28 weeks of gestation when the lentiform nucleus, caudate nucleus, amygdala, hippocampus and the corpus callosum were clearly denoted. This is different from the previous literature showing that the lentiform nucleus and the internal capsule were evident by 11 weeks of gestation, as put forward in one of the figures in that literature [7]. At 28 weeks of gestation, the cortex also showed formation of many new gyri and sulci, in addition to the central sulcus, starting from the middle part of the hemisphere and surrounding areas. This latter trend is similarly observed by Moore and Persaud [7]. The internal capsule was neither morphologically observable nor distinct by MRI until 30 weeks of gestation, at a time when the fornix was also evident. Later, prominent amounts of commissural fibers further crossed over in different bilateral tracts (e.g. anterior commissure). There was a great increase in the volume of white fibers in the medulla of the brain between 30 and 37 weeks of gestation. At birth, the fetal brain was like that of a child, confirming Tilney's [3] gross observations. With advancing imaging technology, it is envisaged that finer observations with superior methods (e.g. in dissecting pathways by imaging) could be achieved [18] in the years to come. Although many of the images at this stage of MRI development are not optimal, mainly due to the movement of the fetus, this paper outlines the important dates in the detailed genesis of the CNS in the living fetus. Based on this study, it is apparent that 25–30 weeks of gestation are crucial in human brain development and this information must be imparted to both students and researchers in the field. This timing is aligned with our previous studies on the histological differentiation of different regions of the human cortex [19].

References

1 Hochstetter F: Beiträge zur Entwicklungsgeschichte des menschlichen Gehirns. Deuticke, Vienna, 1919.
2 Hines M: Studies in the growth and differentiation of the telencephalon in man. The fissura hippocampi. J Comp Neurol 1922;34:73–171.
3 Tilney F: The hippocampus and its relations to the corpus callosum. Bull Neurol Inst NY 1938;7:1–77.
4 Hamilton WJ, Boyd JD, Mossman HW: Human Embryology, ed 2. Cambridge, Heffer, 1959.
5 Yew DT, Lam ST, Liu HC: Development of the human nervous system in fetuses of Chinese descent – from 80 mm (4 month) to 240 mm CR (end of 7 month gestation). Anat Anz 1985;158:343–358.
6 Muller F, O'Rahilly R: The development of the human brain, including the longitudinal zoning in the diencephalon at stage 15. Anat Embryol (Berl) 1988;179:55–71.
7 Moore KL, Persaud TVN: The Developing Human, ed 6. Philadelphia, Saunders, 1998.
8 Takanashi J, Barkovich AJ: The changing MR imaging appearance of polymicrogyria: a consequence of myelination. AJNR Am J Neuroradiol 2003;24:788–793.
9 Fang M, Lorke DE, Li J, Gong X, Yew JC, Yew DT: Postnatal changes in functional activities of the pig's brain: a combined functional magnetic resonance imaging and immunohistochemical study. Neurosignals 2005;14:222–233.
10 Fang M, Li J, Rudd JA, Wai SM, Yew JC, Yew DT: fMRI mapping of cortical centers following visual stimulation in postnatal pigs of different ages. Life Sci 2006;78:1197–1201.
11 D'Incerti L: Morphological neuroimaging of malformations of cortical development. Epileptic Disord 2003;5(suppl 2):S59–S66.
12 Colombo N, Citterio A, Galli C, Tassi L, Lo Russo G, Scialfa G, Spreafico R: Neuroimaging of focal cortical dysplasia: neuropathological correlations. Epileptic Disord 2003; 5(suppl 2):S67–S72.
13 Righini A, Zirpoli S, Mrakic F, Parazzini C, Pogliani L, Triulzi F: Early prenatal MR imaging diagnosis of polymicrogyria. AJNR Am J Neuroradiol 2004;25:343–346.
14 Ghai S, Fong KW, Toi A, Chitayat D, Pantazi S, Blaser S: Prenatal US and MR imaging findings of lissencephaly: review of fetal cerebral sulcal development. Radiographics 2006;26:389–405.
15 Sbarbati A, Pizzini F, Fabene PF, Nicolato E, Marzola P, Calderan L, Simonati A, Longo L, Osculati A, Beltramello A: Cerebral cortex three-dimensional profiling in human fetuses by magnetic resonance imaging. J Anat 2004;204:465–474.
16 Tovar-Moll F, Moll J, de Oliveira-Souza R, Bramati I, Andreiuolo PA, Lent R: Neuroplasticity in human callosal dysgenesis: a diffusion tensor imaging study. Cereb Cortex 2007;17:531–541.
17 Nishida M, Makris N, Kennedy DN, Vangel M, Fischl B, Krishnamoorthy KS, Caviness VS, Grant PE: Detailed semiautomated MRI based morphometry of the neonatal brain: preliminary results. Neuroimage 2006;32:1041–1049.
18 Lee FK, Fang MR, Antonio GE, Yeung DK, Chan ET, Zhang LH, Yew DT, Ahuja AT: Diffusion tensor imaging (DTI) of rodent brains in vivo using a 1.5T clinical MR scanner. J Magn Reson Imaging 2006;23:747–751.
19 Tiu SC, Yew DT, Chan WY: Development of the human cerebral cortex: a histochemical study. Prog Histochem Cytochem 2002;38:3–149.

Neuroembryology and Aging

Neuroembryol Aging 2008;5:39–48
DOI: 10.1159/000116731

Received: October 25, 2007
Accepted: December 19, 2007
Published online: August 19, 2008

Magnetic Resonance Imaging and Its Usage in Representative Areas of Neurobiological Research

A Brief Review

Chun Shi[a, b] W.H. Kwong[a] E. Lucy Forster[a] Eric Y.P. Cho[a]

Departments of Anatomy, [a]Chinese University of Hong Kong, Hong Kong, SAR, and [b]Zhongshan Medical College, Sun Yat Sen University, Guangzhou, China

Key Words
Aging brain · Experimental MRI · Methodologies, MRI · MRI · Neonatal development · Neurobiology

Abstract
This paper summarizes the various methodologies used in magnetic resonance imaging (MRI) and presents the background logic behind these methodologies. The usage of MRI in the study of human subjects and animals is discussed and highlighted. Select examples of animal MR images are presented.

Introduction

Magnetic resonance imaging (MRI) is a noninvasive method of producing highly detailed images of the inside of an object by taking advantage of the magnetic properties of hydrogen and their interaction with both radio waves and an external magnetic field. In its early days, MRI was known as NMR or nuclear MR. Although the name has changed (primarily due to the negative connotation of the word 'nuclear'), the basic principles are the same. Images were derived from the MR properties of hydrogen. Today, MRI is primarily applied in medical imaging to detect pathological and/or physiological alterations of living tissues. It can also be used for nonmedical purposes such as detecting rock permeability to hydrocarbons or characterizing the quality of products such as timber.

History of MRI

The discovery of MRI is one of the most spectacular and successful events in the history of medical imaging. However, there is a huge time gap of almost 30 years between the simultaneous and independent discovery of NMR by Bloch et al. [1] and Purcell et al. [2] in 1946 and the first imaging experiments in the 1970s by Damadian [3].

Since 1950, NMR became an important technique for non-destructive chemical analyses, but interest in the medical diagnostic possibilities of NMR actually began in 1971 with the study by Damadian [3] of the differences in relaxation times T_1 and T_2 between different tissues and between normal and cancerous tissue. Subsequently, the selective slice excitation technique was introduced (an important improvement generally used today) in which a field gradient perpendicular to the selected plane

KARGER

Fax +41 61 306 12 34
E-Mail karger@karger.ch
www.karger.com

1661–3406/08/0052–0039$24.50/0

Accessible online at:
www.karger.com/nba

E. Lucy Forster
Department of Anatomy
Chinese University of Hong Kong
Shatin, N.T., Hong Kong, SAR (China)
Tel. +852 2696 1226, Fax +852 2603 5031, E-Mail lforsterhk@yahoo.com.hk

was applied during a tailored excitation pulse. Through a combination of excitation pulses and orthogonal gradient pulses, a line scan technique was developed by the Mansfield group [4] and was used for the first human whole-body scan in 1978 [5]. In 1975, the 2-dimensional Fourier imaging technique was first applied by Kumar et al. [6] followed by the application of 3-dimensional Fourier images and the production of all the possible cross-sectional images of a selected volume in one scanning procedure. In 1983, Twieg [7] and Ljunggren [8] introduced the trajectory formulation of the MRI process, a very useful tool for the understanding and characterization of the numerous imaging techniques, which has now become a fundamental concept in the analyses of images. Further, improvement in signal detection, fast data handling and gradient technology plus advanced understanding of spin systems, pulse sequences and artifact suppression have greatly shortened the scan time. At present, the most advanced idea in very fast imaging originates from the 'echo-planar' imaging technique proposed by Mansfield [9]. This technique and its derivatives have paved the way for a number of new clinical imaging applications, such as diffusion and perfusion imaging, and functional brain imaging, among others.

Principles of MRI

The basis of MRI is the directional magnetic field, or *moment*, associated with charged particles in motion. Nuclei containing an odd number of protons and neutrons have a characteristic motion or *precession*. Because nuclei are charged particles, this precession produces a small magnetic moment.

When a human body is placed in a magnetic field, many of the free hydrogen nuclei align themselves in the direction of the magnetic field. The nuclei precession about the magnetic field direction is similar to gyroscopic motion. This behavior is termed *Larmor precession*.

The frequency of Larmor precession is proportional to the applied magnetic field strength as defined by the *Larmor frequency*, ω_0:

$$\omega_0 = \gamma B_0 \text{ [10]},$$

where γ is the *gyromagnetic ratio* and B_0 is the strength of the applied magnetic field. The gyromagnetic ratio is a nucleus-specific constant. In the case of protons,

$$\gamma = 42.6 \times 10^6 \text{ MHz/T [10]}.$$

To obtain an MR image of an object, the object is placed in a uniform magnetic field, B_0, of 0.5–1.5 T. As a result, the object's hydrogen nuclei align with the magnetic field and create a net magnetic moment, M, parallel to B_0. Next, a radiofrequency (RF) pulse, B_{rf}, is applied perpendicular to B_0. This pulse, with a frequency equal to the Larmor frequency, causes M to tilt away from B_0.

Once the RF signal is removed, the nuclei realign themselves such that their net magnetic moment, M, is again parallel to B_0. This return to equilibrium is referred to as *relaxation*. During relaxation, the nuclei lose energy by emitting their own RF signal. This signal is referred to as the *free-induction decay* (FID) response signal. The FID response signal is measured by a conductive field coil placed around the object being imaged. This measurement is processed or *reconstructed* to obtain 3D gray-scale MR images.

To produce a 3D image, the FID resonance signal must be encoded for each dimension. The encoding in the axial direction, the direction of B_0, is accomplished by adding a gradient magnetic field to B_0. This gradient causes the Larmor frequency to change linearly in the axial direction. Thus, an axial slice can be selected by choosing the frequency of the RF pulse, B_{rf}, to correspond to the Larmor frequency of that slice. The 2D spatial reconstruction in each axial slice is accomplished using frequency and phase encoding. A 'preparation' gradient, G_y, is applied causing the resonant frequencies of the nuclei to vary according to their position in the y-direction. G_y is then removed and another gradient, G_x, is applied perpendicular to G_y. As a result, the resonant frequencies of the nuclei vary in the x-direction due to G_x and have a phase variation in the y-direction due to the previously applied G_y. Thus, x-direction samples are encoded by frequency and y-direction samples are encoded by phase. A 2D Fourier Transform is then used to transform the encoded image to the spatial domain.

The voxel (volume picture elements) intensity of a given tissue type (i.e. white vs. gray matter) depends on the *proton density* of the tissue; the higher the proton density, the stronger the FID response signal. MR image contrast also depends on two other tissue-specific parameters: the longitudinal relaxation time, 'Time 1' or T_1, and the transverse relaxation time, 'Time 2' or T_2. T_1 represents the time required for the magnetic moment of the displaced nuclei to return to equilibrium. T_2 indicates the time required for the FID response signal from a given tissue type to decay.

When MR images are acquired, the RF pulse, B_{rf}, is repeated at a predetermined rate. The period of the RF pulse sequence is the *repetition time*, *TR*. The FID response signals can be measured at various times within the *TR* interval. The time between which the RF pulse is applied and the response signal measured is the *echo delay time*, *TE*. By adjusting *TR* and *TE*, the acquired MR image can be made to contrast different tissue types.

System Architecture

A static magnetic field, an RF transmitter and receiver, and three orthogonal, controllable magnetic gradients form the major components of an MRI scanner.

Magnets

A constant magnetic field is generated by magnets. Magnets, either electric current conducting (electromagnet) or permanent magnetic (ferromagnetic) material, are the most important components of the scanner. The straightness of magnetic lines within the center or the isocenter of the magnet needs to be almost perfect. This is known as homogeneity. Fluctuations or non-homogeneities in the field strength within the scan region should be less than 3 ppm. There are three basic types of magnets used in MRI systems: resistive, permanent and superconducting magnets.

Resistive Magnets. Resistive magnets consist of many windings or coils of wire wrapped around a cylinder or bore, through which an electric current is passed to generate a magnetic field. This kind of magnet is lower in cost than a superconducting magnet but requires huge amounts of electricity (up to 50 kW) to operate because of the natural resistance in the wire.

Permanent Magnets. A permanent magnet is a conventional magnet made from ferromagnetic material such as steel. Its magnetic field is permanent and always on full strength. The major drawback is that this magnet is extremely heavy and can achieve only limited field strength (<0.4 T), with limited stability and precision. There are also potential safety issues, as the magnetic field cannot be removed in case of entrapment.

Superconducting Magnets. A superconducting magnet is somewhat similar to a resistive magnet: coils or windings of wire through which an electric current is passed create the magnetic field. The important difference is that the wire is continually bathed in liquid helium at –267.77°C to cause the resistance in the wire to reach zero, dramatically reducing the electrical requirement of the system and making it much more economical to operate. Moreover, it is well insulated by a vacuum in a manner identical to that used in a vacuum flask. Superconductive systems are very expensive, but they can easily generate 0.5- to 2.0-tesla fields, allowing for much higher-quality imaging, therefore superconducting magnets are the most common type found in MRI scanners today.

Magnetic field strength is an important factor determining image quality. Higher magnetic fields increase the signal-to-noise ratio, permitting higher resolution or faster scanning. However, higher field strengths require more costly magnets with higher maintenance costs, and have increased safety concerns. The 1.0- to 1.5-tesla field strengths are a good compromise between cost and performance for general medical use. However, for certain specific uses such as brain imaging, field strengths up to 3.0 T may be desirable.

The Radiofrequency Chain

The RF chain consists of the transmitting part and the receiving part. The transmitting chain starts with the frequency synthesizer, followed by the amplitude modulator. The signal from the amplitude modulator is fed into the power amplifier. The amplifier is capable of delivering a peak RF power of 5–23 kW. When the power amplifier is active, it is connected to the transmitting coil (a large coil having a major region with a homogenous RF magnetic field). This is desirable for homogeneous slice excitation. During transmission, all 'receive-only' coils are open circuited to prevent the transmitting power from entering the receiving system. When the power amplifier is not active, its output is disconnected in order to prevent its output noise from interfering with the small signals in the system. Also during reception, the transmitting coil is open circuited with a switch to avoid mutual couplings with the receive coils.

The receive chain starts with the receiving coil, which is tuned to the signal frequency. In the coil, a first-amplifier stage is integrated to avoid signal loss due to the cable between the coil and the receiver. Then the signal is again amplified and subsequently digitized in an analog-to-digital converter. The signal is in a form that can be fed into the Fourier transformer, which must be a rapid circuit to make images available within a second after the scan is completed.

The Gradient Chain

Gradient fields are added to the main magnetic field to position encode the signal emitted by the proton spins in the object. These gradient fields are generated with three orthogonal coils, oriented in the x, y and z directions of the scanner. Usually, a gradient system can produce gradients from 20 to 100 mT/m. As the orthogonal gradients can be combined freely, any plane can be selected for imaging.

Contrast Enhancement

As mentioned above, contrast in MRI is the difference between two signal levels in adjacent tissue regions, which depends on relaxation times T_1 and T_2, the proton density of the tissues and the sequence parameters. Both T_1- and T_2-weighted images are required in most medical examinations. However, the anatomy or pathology is sometimes not adequately shown. The need to more accurately characterize different types of lesions and to detect all malignant lesions are the main reasons for the use of more sophisticated image acquisition techniques (e.g. fat suppression or chemical-shift imaging [11]) and the use of intravenous contrast agents.

There are some methods to improve the contrast of different tissues: *dynamic contrast-enhanced MRI* focuses on contrast kinetics with demands for spatial resolution dependent on the application; it is mainly used for diagnosis of cancer and cardiac infarction. *Contrast-enhanced MR angiography* (MRA) allows the visualization of vessels with temporal resolution to provide a separation of arteries and veins. Double contrast administration *(combined contrast-enhanced MRI)* uses two contrast agents with complementary mechanisms in, for example, superparamagnetic iron oxide to darken the background liver and gadolinium to brighten the vessels. A variety of different categories of contrast agents are currently available for clinical use.

Advantages of MRI and Its Clinical Applications

The major technological advantage of MRI is that it can characterize and discriminate between tissues using their physical and biochemical properties (water, iron, fat, and extravascular blood and its breakdown products). Blood flow, cerebrospinal fluid flow, and contraction and relaxation of organs, both physiologic and pathologic, can be evaluated. Because calcium emits no signal on spin echo images, beam-hardening artifacts can be avoided and tissues surrounded by bone can be imaged, such as the contents of the posterior fossa and the spine. Moreover, MRI produces sectional images of equivalent resolution in any projection without moving the patient. This ability to obtain images in multiple planes offers special advantages for radiation and surgical treatment planning. In addition, MR image acquisition does not use ionizing radiation or iodinated contrast agents. Para- and superparamagnetic contrast agents that appear to be relatively nontoxic permit evaluation of the integrity of the blood-brain barrier, the reticulo-endothelial system and the extracellular space.

Therefore, the noninvasive MRI technique is ideal for:

- diagnosing infections in the brain, spine or joints;
- visualizing torn ligaments in the wrist, knee and ankle;
- visualizing shoulder injuries;
- diagnosing tendonitis;
- evaluating masses in the soft tissues of the body;
- evaluating bone tumors, cysts, and bulging or herniated vertebral discs;
- diagnosing strokes in their earliest stages;
- diagnosing multiple sclerosis, and
- diagnosing tumors of the pituitary gland and brain.

Limitations

The relatively slow scan acquisition time results in artifacts due to biological (physiological) motion, e.g. cardiac, vascular or cerebrospinal fluid pulsation, respiratory excursion and gastrointestinal peristalsis. Technological advances such as cine MRI, improved surface coils, respiratory, cardiac and peripheral gating, chemical shift imaging and fast scanning (gradient refocused images) may resolve many of these problems. Because of the small bore of the magnet, some patients experience claustrophobia and have difficulty cooperating during the study. Severely obese patients cannot be examined because they cannot fit into most MRI machines, although there are some larger-bore machines being developed. Patients with pacemakers and ferromagnetic appliances usually cannot be assessed, although new pacemakers and implanted defibrillators have been designed to cope with this issue.

Although the appearance of calcium as a signal void provides some advantages, it also limits the ability to detect pathological calcification in soft tissues and tumors, and pathological changes in cortical bone are poorly depicted with routine spin echo techniques. Other imaging sequences may permit visualization of some of these lesions.

Presently, contrast agents to enhance the MR images are not approved for general use in the United States. There has also been some recent concern that administration of gadolinium-based contrast agents to patients with renal diseases increases the risk of nephrogenic systemic fibrosis [12], and the US Food and Drug Administration has issued a warning statement about it. Greater technological expertise is required for utilization of MRI than for most other imaging techniques. These factors limit the present application of MRI.

Specialized MRI Scans

Functional MRI

The principle of functional MRI (fMRI) is based on the increase in blood flow in the local vasculature that accompanies neural activity in the brain, resulting in a corresponding local reduction in deoxyhemoglobin because the increase in blood flow occurs without an increase in similar magnitude in oxygen extraction [13–16]. Since deoxyhemoglobin is paramagnetic, it alters the T_2-weighted MR image signal [17–23]. Using an appropriate imaging sequence, human cortical functions can be observed [24–28]. Functional activity of the brain determined from the MR signal has confirmed known anatomically distinct processing areas in the visual cortex [19, 28–33], the motor cortex [34, 35] and in Broca's area of speech and language-related activities [36, 37]. Further, much literature reports corresponding findings between fMRI and conventional electrophysiological techniques to localize specific functions of the human brain [38–44].

Using fMRI to image brain activity related to a specific task or sensory process has many advantages, for example, the signal does not require injections of radioactive isotopes, the total scan time required can be very short and the in-plane resolution of the functional image is generally about 1.5×1.5 mm, although resolutions <1 mm are possible. Putting these advantages in perspective, fMRI will have many new neuroscience applications.

Diffusion MRI

Another very revealing MRI method is 'diffusion tensor MRI', known as DT-MRI or DTI [45]. The technology evaluates the random motion of hydrogen atoms in water molecules, noninvasively, in vivo and in three dimensions, thus implementing the phenomenon of diffusion. High-speed collision of molecules causes water to 'diffuse' out in different speeds in different directions, thus establishing a pattern for different cells and tissues. More specifically, image intensities at each position are attenuated, depending on the strength (b-value) and direction of the so-called magnetic diffusion gradient, as well as on the local microstructure in which the water molecules diffuse. The more attenuated the image is at a given position, the more diffusion there is in the direction of the diffusion gradient.

Traditionally, in diffusion-weighted imaging (DWI), three gradient directions are applied, sufficient to estimate the trace of the diffusion tensor or 'average diffusivity', a putative measure of edema. Clinically, trace-weighted images have proven very useful in the diagnosis of vascular strokes in the brain by early detection (within 6 h) of hypoxic edema [46], although some lesions are better detected by computer tomography (CT) scans [47].

More extended DTI scans comprise at least six gradient directions, sufficient to compute the diffusion tensor. From the diffusion tensor, diffusion anisotropy measures, such as the fractional anisotropy, can be computed. Moreover, the principal direction of the diffusion tensor can be used to infer the white-matter connectivity of the brain (i.e. tractography, or to determine which part of the brain is connected to which other part).

Recently, more advanced models of the diffusion process have been proposed that aim to overcome the weaknesses of the diffusion tensor model. Among others, these include q-space imaging and generalized DTI.

Magnetic Resonance Angiography

MR angiography (MRA) is a medical imaging technique used to visualize blood-filled structures, including arteries, veins and the heart chambers. This MRI technique creates soft tissue contrast between blood vessels and surrounding tissues primarily by visualizing blood flow within the vessels, rather than by displaying the vessel lumen. There are bright blood and black blood MRA techniques, named according to the appearance of the blood vessels. Contrast-enhanced MRA creates the angiographic effect by using an intravenously administered MR contrast agent to selectively shorten the T_1 of blood and thereby cause the vessels to appear bright on T_1-weighted images.

MRA is often used to evaluate the arteries of the neck and brain, the thoracic and abdominal aorta, the renal arteries, and the legs for stenosis or aneurysms.

Magnetic Resonance Spectroscopy

MR spectroscopic imaging (MRS/MRSI) is a method using the NMR phenomenon to identify the chemical state of various elements without destroying the sample. The underlying principle of MRS is that atomic nuclei are surrounded by a cloud of electrons slightly shielding the nucleus from any external magnetic field. Since the structure of the electron cloud is specific to an individual molecule or compound, the magnitude of this screening effect is also characteristic of the chemical environment of individual nuclei. MRS thereby provides information about the chemical composition of the tissues and the changes in chemical composition, which may occur with disease processes.

Interventional MRI

An increasing number of interventional procedures are done under imaging guidance. These include biopsies, fluid drainages and injections. Likewise, imaging guidance and monitoring have enabled the use of sophisticated techniques for minimally invasive therapy of tumors. Since MRI provides the best tissue contrast and lesion sensitivity, the use of MR-guided procedures is quickly gaining momentum. Special hardware and software solutions have been developed that allow more efficient interventional use of the MR scanner.

Radiation Therapy Simulation

MRI is used routinely for radiation therapy simulation now because of its superior imaging of soft tissue. During radiation therapy simulation, the MRI unit can compute the accurate location, shape and orientation of tumors within the body, correcting for any spatial distortion inherent in the system. Open MRI is reported to be temporally stable and to have sufficient geometric accuracy for most radiation therapy planning [48].

Current Density Imaging

Current density imaging is an imaging technique that measures electrical current density vectors in a volume of material/tissue that can be imaged using MRI. Measurements are performed by applying an external current to the material and/or tissue during MRI acquisition. The magnetic fields produced by the applied current are mapped onto the phase images of the MRI acquisition. The phase images are processed to reconstruct current densities within a subject.

Magnetic Resonance-Guided Focused Ultrasound

MR-guided focused ultrasound is often shortened to MRgFUS. MRI is used to identify tumors or fibroids in the body before they are destroyed by ultrasound. MRgFUS is currently used in the US, Canada, Israel, Europe and Asia to treat uterine fibroids. Current clinical trials are underway examining the possible use of the technique in the treatment of cancers of the brain, breast, liver, bone and prostate.

Multinuclear Imaging

With the use of specially designed multiple-tuned probes for MRI, multinuclear imaging was developed which enabled us to obtain images of different nuclei simultaneously. Both phantom and in vivo MR images of two nuclei (e.g. hydrogen-1, phosphorus-31, lithium-7 or fluorine-19) were obtained in the time span necessary to collect the image of the less sensitive nuclei. This technique offers a means to gather physiological and anatomical information in a highly efficient manner [49].

Multinuclear imaging is primarily used as a research technique at present. Inhaled hyperpolarized ^{3}He can be used to image the distribution of air spaces within the lungs. Injectable solutions containing ^{13}C or stabilized bubbles of hyperpolarized ^{129}Xe have been studied as contrast agents for angiography and perfusion imaging. ^{31}P can potentially provide information on bone density and structure, as well as functional imaging of the brain.

Other Experimental MRI Techniques

Currently, several new MRI technologies such as magnetization transfer MRI, DT-MRI (DTI), proton MRS and dendrimer-enhanced MRI are in active research and may provide more anatomic, physiologic and pharmacologic information in future medical imaging.

Future of MRI

MRI is not only effective for the detection and localization of tissue, but also offers promise for tissue characterization. Future applications of MRI may include nonproton imaging, e.g. phosphorus and sodium. The combination of imaging with localized in vivo spectroscopy may reveal fundamental information regarding the metabolic status of a particular organ or lesion. The phosphorus metabolite concentration, for example, may be measurable as a reflection of the state of oxygenation of the myocardium or of tumors. However, the application of MRI to the vascular system needs further exploration. It may be employed as a noninvasive means of assessing peripheral venous disease.

Gadolinium diethylenetriamine penta-acetic acid is one of the contrast agents used with MRI. Paramagnetic-labeled pharmaceuticals and monoclonal antibodies offer more opportunities for acquiring anatomic, physiologic and pharmacologic information. With the use of such agents, disorders characterized by qualitatively or quantitatively abnormal receptor sites could be documented more conclusively.

So far, MRI has been considered as a safe modality for imaging. Nevertheless, there must be further investigation of its secondary effects, such as local heating of tissues. The potential somatic and genetic effects of MR also need continued investigation to confirm its safety.

Applications of MRI

Usage in Neurobiological Research

MRI is now routinely used in neurological research, particularly in morphological and experimental studies, to reveal both anticipated and de novo results. In the early 1990s, bilateral carotid artery occlusions of cats in the 2nd postnatal week were performed in experimental studies with unexpected outcomes. MRI observation, along with histological studies, reported cell death in the motor cortex while the visual cortex showed an increased number of neurons, with thinning of the corpus callosum, in the experimental animals [50]. Other work in the '90s employed freezing injury to the cortex, subsequently observed by MRI and histology [51]. Often however, especially in the early MRI studies, the resolution and contrast appeared marginal, so various contrasting agents were proposed to reduce this problem. Lately, for example, in a study of the cerebellum of the neonatal mouse, manganese enhancement was performed, and the granule cells appeared to show substantial uptake of the metal, giving a high contrast in MR images [52], yet this uptake was not equal among all the cells of different cortical regions. In studies of morphological changes in the nervous system, whether developmental or pathological conditions, the usage of plain MRI in the experienced eye can still reflect subtotal changes. However, in these studies, particularly in animal research, it is always advisable to confirm MRI changes with histology [53]. This is necessary to erase any artifact or overconfidence in interpretation.

Usage in Developmental Neurobiology

Plain MRI studies have been utilized in human studies of the developing brain, from children to adolescents. In the normal young human brain, increases in white matter volume and other regional changes in gray matter have been documented [54]. In children with autism, an abnormal increase in white matter volume has often been associated with poor motor skills in behavioral tests [55]. Such increases in white matter as seen by MRI have also been found in the brains of schizophrenic patients and their relatives, which may be the result of dysmyelination between the stages of adolescence and adulthood [56]. Effects of prenatal maternal intake of drugs on the fetal or neonatal brain (whether of abusive agents or potentially damaging therapeutic drugs) have been outlined by MRI by quantitation of gray matter in the basal ganglia, hypothalamus and the frontal cortex [57–59]. It is thus evident that the use of MRI in studies of the brains of living animals and humans has gained popularity in scientific research. In addition, MRI has also been utilized in fixed tissue specimens of the mouse brain and has been found satisfactory for observation [60].

While simple MRI studies have been efficacious, its uses in developmental research are still limited. MRI studies have been done in the developing ferret brain to identify cortical gyrus formation. It was concluded that MRI revealed major cortical folding completed prior to myelination of deeper white fibers in these animals [61]. MRI has been suggested for use in tracing of stem cell migration [62]. Although this has great potential in research, such studies are only useful in animals where tracers can be used. In studies in humans, tracers or contrast media have not been allowed as they might pass through the placenta [63]. Further, despite the absence of deleterious MRI effects on pregnancy, thus far MRI usage is limited to the second and third trimesters [63] in pregnancy.

DTI has been found useful for studying brain pathology [64] and the development of the cortical plate and axonal tracts in the normal mouse or rat [65–67] and the mutant mouse [68]. In the latter study, for example, axonal growth in the default pathways of the mutant frizzled 3 mice was determined by this technique [68].

While no thorough DTI study of the human brain has been conducted to date, two very interesting works have been performed in this area. The first work utilized fetal specimens aged 31–37 weeks where DTI reported a significant age increase in apparent diffusion coefficient and fractional anisotropy in the pyramidal tract and corpus callosum [69]. The second more recent DTI study [70] of the brainstem, cerebellum and thalamus in 23- to 37-week-old fetuses reported a negative linear correlation of the diffusion coefficient with gestational age. In the supratentorial area, an increase was detected in the apparent diffusion coefficient values at 30 weeks of gestation [70]. Although information gained from DTI has been useful in studies of tracts, for example, using DTI with fixed baboon brains from 90 to 185 gestational days [71], there is limited information on the gray matter during brain development.

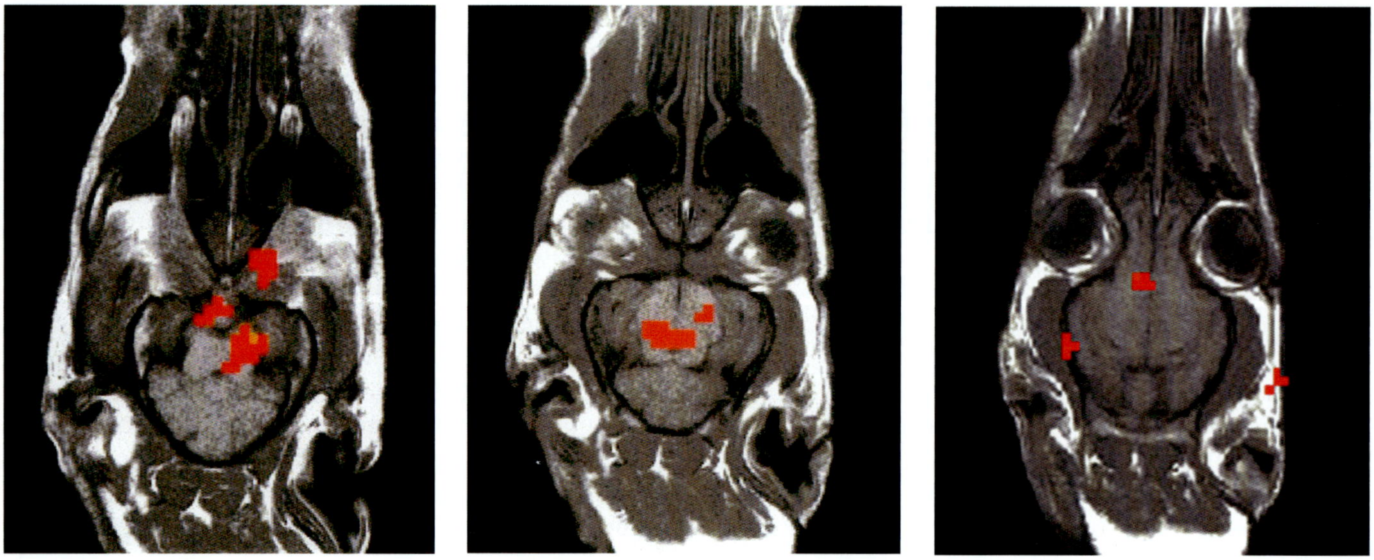

Fig. 1–3. fMR images of 1- (**1**), 2- (**2**) and 3-month-old pig brainstem (**3**) upon stimulation.

Morphological studies have not always yielded all the answers. fMRI can provide additional information by analyzing blood oxygen activities to show changes in brain function. fMRI studies have been very informative in the field of plasticity and development [72], yet are currently limited in the prenatal environment as fMRI usually requires certain types of stimuli for data analysis. For research of neonatal development and aging, a number of studies have been performed in the pig and mouse [53, 67, 73–77] (fig. 1–3). In the neonatal pig, a study of the development of motor and sensory activities via motor or sensory or both stimuli reported that the cortex would not be totally mature until 6 months postnatally [75, 77]. Initially, a small stimulus might result in an overreaction of many parts of the cortex but subsequently showed maturation through an increase in inhibitory control [75]. This is also true for the visual pathways controlling color vision in that these pathways do not appear to be fully functional until 6 months after birth [77]. fMRI has also been used for research involving subjects with 22q11.2 deletion syndrome that affects the catechol-O-methyltransferase gene. Irregular cingulate activities have been observed when subjects went through attention and inhibition testing [78].

Another recently developed imaging system, proton MRS or ^{1}H-MRS, uses the photon spectrum to show peaks for levels of N-acetylaspartate, choline compounds, creatine and other common brain metabolites. Research using ^{1}H-MRS can observe changes due to altered metabolic states, e.g. after prenatal cocaine exposure, creatine elevation was noted in the frontal areas of the exposed children [79]. In the future, the study of these metabolic states in the developing fetus would be very useful to understand normal and abnormal changes in morphogenesis.

Conclusion

In summary, with the introduction of the various approaches in MRI, studies of the functional and metabolic states in the living brain are no longer out of reach. These techniques are vitally useful in experimental and clinical neurology, and in research to decipher changes and mechanisms of changes in the developing and aging brain.

References

1 Bloch F, Hansen WW, Packard M: Nuclear induction. Phys Rev 1946;69:127.
2 Purcell EM, Torrey HC, Pound RV: Resonance absorption by nuclear magnetic moments in a solid. Phys Rev 1946;69:37–38.
3 Damadian R: Tumor detection by nuclear magnetic resonance. Science 1971;171:1151–1153.
4 Mansfield P, Maudsley AA: Line scan proton spin imaging in biological structures by NMR. Phys Med Biol 1976;21:847–852.
5 Mansfield P, Pykett IL, Morris PG: Human whole body line-scan imaging by NMR. Br J Radiol 1978;51:921–922.

6 Kumar A, Welti D, Ernst RR: NMR Fourier zeugmatography. J Magn Reson 1975;18:69–83.
7 Twieg D: The k-trajectory formulation of the NMR imaging process with applications in analysis and synthesis of imaging methods. Med Phys 1983;10:610–621.
8 Ljunggren S: A simple graphical representation of Fourier-based imaging methods. J Magn Reson 1983;54:338–343.
9 Mansfield P: Multiplanar image formation using NMR spin echoes. J Phys C Solid State Phys 1977;10:L55–L58.
10 Vlaardingerbroek MT, den Boer JA: Magnetic Resonance Imaging: Theory and Practice, ed 3. Berlin, Springer, 2003, p 10.
11 Haase A, Frahm J, Hänicke W, Matthaei D: ^{1}H NMR chemical shift selective (CHESS) imaging. Phys Med Biol 1985;30:341–344.
12 Grobner T: Gadolinium – a specific trigger for the development of nephrogenic fibrosing dermopathy and nephrogenic systemic fibrosis? Nephrol Dial Transplant 2006;21:1104–1108.
13 Roy C, Sherrington C: On the regulation of the blood supply of the brain. J Physiol 1890;11:85–108.
14 Plum F, Posner JB, Troy B: Cerebral metabolic and circulatory responses to induced convulsions in animals. Arch Neurol 1968;18:1–13.
15 Posner JB, Plum F, Van Poznak A: Cerebral metabolism during electrically induced seizures in man. Arch Neurol 1969;20:388–395.
16 Fox PT, Raichle ME: Stimulus rate determines regional brain blood flow in striate cortex. Ann Neurol 1985;17:303–305.
17 Ogawa S, Lee TM, Nayak AS, Glynn P: Oxygenation-sensitive contrast in magnetic resonance image of rodent brain at high magnetic fields. Magn Reson Med 1990;14:68–78.
18 Ogawa S, Lee TM, Kay AR, Tank DW: Brain magnetic resonance imaging with contrast dependent on blood oxygenation. Proc Natl Acad Sci USA 1990;87:9868–9872.
19 Ogawa S, Tank DW, Menon R, Ellermann JM, Kim SG, Merkle H, Ugurbil K: Intrinsic signal changes accompanying sensory stimulation: functional brain mapping with magnetic resonance imaging. Proc Natl Acad Sci USA 1992;89:5951–5955.
20 Ogawa S, Menon RS, Tank DW, Kim SG, Merkle H, Ellermann JM, Ugurbil K: Functional brain mapping by blood oxygenation level-dependent contrast magnetic resonance imaging. A comparison of signal characteristics with a biophysical model. Biophys J 1993;64:803–812.
21 Belliveau JW, Rosen BR, Kantor HL, Rzedzian RR, Kennedy DN, McKinstry RC, Vevea JM, Cohen MS, Pykett IL, Brady TJ: Functional cerebral imaging by susceptibility-contrast NMR. Magn Reson Med 1990;14:538–546.
22 Turner R, Le Bihan D, Moonen CT, Despres D, Frank J: Echo-planar time course MRI of cat brain oxygenation changes. Magn Reson Med 1991;22:159–166.
23 Tank DW, Ogawa S, Ugurbil K: Mapping the brain with MRI. Curr Biol 1992;2:525–528.
24 Bandettini PA, Wong EC, Hinks RS, Tikofsky RS, Hyde JS: Time course EPI of human brain function during task activation. Magn Reson Med 1992;25:390–397.
25 Bandettini PA, Jesmanowicz A, Wong EC, Hyde JS: Processing strategies for time-course data sets in functional MRI of the human brain. Magn Reson Med 1993;30:161–173.
26 Kwong KK, Belliveau JW, Chesler DA, Goldberg IE, Weisskoff RM, Poncelet BP, Kennedy DN, Hoppel BE, Cohen MS, Turner R, Cheng HM, Brady TJ, Rosen BR: Dynamic magnetic resonance imaging of human brain activity during primary sensory stimulation. Proc Natl Acad Sci USA 1992;89:5675–5679.
27 Turner R, Jezzard P, Wen H, Kwong KK, Le Bihan D, Zeffiro T, Balaban RS: Functional mapping of the human visual cortex at 4 and 1.5 tesla using deoxygenation contrast EPI. Magn Reson Med 1993;29:277–279.
28 Schneider W, Noll DC, Cohen JD: Functional topographic mapping of the cortical ribbon in human vision with conventional MRI scanners. Nature 1993;365:150–153.
29 Belliveau JW, Kennedy DN Jr, McKinstry RC, Buchbinder BR, Weisskoff RM, Cohen MS, Vevea JM, Brady TJ, Rosen BR: Functional mapping of the human visual cortex by magnetic resonance imaging. Science 1991;254:716–719.
30 Blamire AM, Ogawa S, Ugurbil K, Rothman D, McCarthy G, Ellermann JM, Hyder F, Rattner Z, Shulman RG: Dynamic mapping of the human visual cortex by high-speed magnetic resonance imaging. Proc Natl Acad Sci USA 1992;89:11069–11073.
31 Hirsch J, DeLaPaz RL, Relkin NR, Victor J, Kim K, Li T, Borden P, Rubin N, Shapley R: Illusory contours activate specific regions in human visual cortex: evidence from functional magnetic resonance imaging. Proc Natl Acad Sci USA 1995;92:6469–6473.
32 Hirsch J, DeLaPaz R, Relkin N, Victor J, Li T, Kim K, Borden P, Lee KM, Rubin N, Shapley R: Human visual processes involved in stereo and illusory contour-defined images are predominantly located in right occipital cortex using functional magnetic resonance imaging (fMRI). Abstr Soc Neurosci 1995;21:18.
33 Hirsch J, DeLaPaz R, Relkin N, Victor J, Li T, Kim K, Rubin N, Shapley R: A study of illusory contours in human cerebral cortex with functional magnetic resonance imaging (fMRI). Invest Ophthalmol Vis Sci 1995;36(suppl):S1068.
34 Kim SG, Ashe J, Georgopoulos AP, Merkle H, Ellermann JM, Menon RS, Ogawa S, Ugurbil K: Functional imaging of human motor cortex at high magnetic field. J Neurophysiol 1993;69:297–302.
35 Kim SG, Ashe J, Hendrich K, Ellermann JM, Merkle H, Uğurbil K, Georgopoulos AP: Functional magnetic resonance imaging of motor cortex: hemispheric asymmetry and handedness. Science 1993;261:615–617.
36 Hinke RM, Hu X, Stillman AE, Kim SG, Merkle H, Salmi R, Ugurbil K: Functional magnetic resonance imaging of Broca's area during internal speech. Neuroreport 1993;4:675–678.
37 Kim K, Hirsch J, DeLaPaz RL, Relkin N, Lee KM: Comparison of cortical areas activated by primary and secondary languages in human brain using functional magnetic resonance imaging (fMRI). Abstr Soc Neurosci 1995;21:1763.
38 Atlas SW, Howard RS 2nd, Maldjian J, Alsop D, Detre JA, Listerud J, D'Esposito M, Judy KD, Zager E, Stecker M: Functional magnetic resonance imaging of regional brain activity in patients with intracerebral gliomas: findings and implications for clinical management. Neurosurgery 1996;38:329–338.
39 Puce A: Comparative assessment of sensorimotor function using functional magnetic resonance imaging and electrophysiological methods. J Clin Neurophysiol 1995;12:450–459.
40 Puce A, Constable RT, Luby ML, McCarthy G, Nobre AC, Spencer DD, Gore JC, Allison T: Functional magnetic resonance imaging of sensory and motor cortex: comparison with electrophysiological localization. J Neurosurg 1995;83:262–270.
41 Burgess RC: Editorial: functional localization by neurophysiologic and neuroimaging techniques. J Clin Neurophysiol 1995;12:405–431.
42 Detre JA, Sirven JI, Alsop DC, O'Connor MJ, French JA: Localization of subclinical ictal activity by functional magnetic resonance imaging: correlation with invasive monitoring. Ann Neurol 1995;38:618–624.
43 George JS, Aine CJ, Mosher JC, Schmidt DM, Ranken DM, Schlitt HA, Wood CC, Lewine JD, Sanders JA, Belliveau JW: Mapping function in the human brain with magnetoencephalography, anatomical magnetic resonance imaging, and functional magnetic resonance imaging. J Clin Neurophysiol 1995;12:406–431.
44 Ives JR, Warach S, Schmitt F, Edelman RR, Schomer DL: Monitoring the patient's EEG during echo planar MRI. Electroencephalogr Clin Neurophysiol 1993;87:417–420.
45 Basser PJ, Mattiello J, LeBihan D: MR diffusion tensor spectroscopy and imaging. Biophys J 1994;66:259–267.
46 Schaefer PW, Copen WA, Lev MH, Gonzalez RG: Diffusion-weighted imaging in acute stroke. Magn Reson Imaging Clin N Am 2006;14:141–168.

47 Kim EY, Ryoo JW, Roh HG, Lee KH, Kim SS, Song IC, Chang KH, Na DG: Reversed discrepancy between CT and diffusion-weighted MR imaging in acute ischemic stroke. AJNR Am J Neuroradiol 2006;27:1990–1995.
48 Mah D, Steckner M, Palacio E, Mitra R, Richardson T, Hanks GE: Characteristics and quality assurance of a dedicated open 0.23 T MRI for radiation therapy simulation. Med Phys 2002;29:2541–2547.
49 Schnall MD, Bolinger L, Renshaw PF, Haselgrove JC, Subramanian VH, Eleff SM, Barlow C, Leigh JS Jr, Chance B: Multinuclear MR imaging: a technique for combined anatomic and physiologic studies. Radiology 1987;162:863–866.
50 Miller B, Nagy D, Finlay BL, Chance B, Kobayashi A, Nioka S: Consequences of reduced cerebral blood flow in brain development. I. Gross morphology, histology, and callosal connectivity. Exp Neurol 1993;124:326–342.
51 Rosen GD, Burstein D: MRI visualization of focal induced neocortical malformations of the rat. Neuroreport 1997;8:3883–3887.
52 Wadghiri YZ, Blind JA, Duan X, Moreno C, Yu X, Joyner AL, Turnbull DH: Manganese-enhanced magnetic resonance imaging (MEMRI) of mouse brain development. NMR Biomed 2004;17:613–619.
53 Fang M, Li J, Gong X, Antonio G, Lee F, Kwong WH, Wai SM, Yew DT: Myelination of the pig's brain: a correlated MRI and histological study. Neurosignals 2005;14:102–108.
54 Lenroot RK, Giedd JN: Brain development in children and adolescents: insights from anatomical magnetic resonance imaging. Neurosci Biobehav Rev 2006;30:718–729.
55 Mostofsky SH, Burgess MP, Gidley Larson JC: Increased motor cortex white matter volume predicts motor impairment in autism. Brain 2007;130:2117–2122.
56 Ho BC: MRI brain volume abnormalities in young, nonpsychotic relatives of schizophrenia probands are associated with subsequent prodromal symptoms. Schizophr Res 2007;96:1–13.
57 Ikonomidou C, Scheer I, Wilhelm T, Juengling FD, Titze K, Stöver B, Lehmkuhl U, Koch S, Kassubek J: Brain morphology alterations in the basal ganglia and the hypothalamus following prenatal exposure to antiepileptic drugs. Eur J Paediatr Neurol 2007;11:297–301.
58 Avants BB, Hurt H, Giannetta JM, Epstein CL, Shera DM, Rao H, Wang J, Gee JC: Effects of heavy in utero cocaine exposure on adolescent caudate morphology. Pediatr Neurol 2007;37:275–279.
59 Sowell ER, Mattson SN, Kan E, Thompson PM, Riley EP, Toga AW: Abnormal cortical thickness and brain-behavior correlation patterns in individuals with heavy prenatal alcohol exposure. Cereb Cortex 2008;18:136–144.
60 Ma Y, Hof PR, Grant SC, Blackband SJ, Bennett R, Slatest L, McGuigan MD, Benveniste H: A three-dimensional digital atlas database of the adult C57BL/6J mouse brain by magnetic resonance microscopy. Neuroscience 2005;135:1203–1215.
61 Neal J, Takahashi M, Silva M, Tiao G, Walsh CA, Sheen VL: Insights into the gyrification of developing ferret brain by magnetic resonance imaging. J Anat 2007;210:66–77.
62 Magnitsky S, Walton RM, Wolfe JH, Poptani H: Magnetic resonance imaging as a tool for monitoring stem cell migration. Neurodegener Dis 2007;4:314–321.
63 Huisman TA, Martin E, Kubik-Huch R, Marincek B: Fetal magnetic resonance imaging of the brain: technical considerations and normal brain development. Eur Radiol 2002;12:1941–1951.
64 Mascalchi M, Filippi M, Floris R, Fonda C, Gasparotti R, Villari N: Diffusion-weighted MR of the brain: methodology and clinical application. Radiol Med (Torino) 2005;109:155–197.
65 Mori S, Itoh R, Zhang J, Kaufmann WE, van Zijl PC, Solaiyappan M, Yarowsky P: Diffusion tensor imaging of the developing mouse brain. Magn Reson Med 2001;46:18–23.
66 Zhang J, Miller MI, Plachez C, Richards LJ, Yarowsky P, van Zijl P, Mori S: Mapping postnatal mouse brain development with diffusion tensor microimaging. Neuroimage 2005;26:1042–1051.
67 Lee FK, Fang MR, Antonio GE, Yeung DK, Chan ET, Zhang LH, Yew DT, Ahuja AT: Diffusion tensor imaging (DTI) of rodent brains in vivo using a 1.5 T clinical MR scanner. J Magn Reson Imaging 2006;23:747–751.
68 Wang Y, Zhang J, Mori S, Nathans J: Axonal growth and guidance defects in Frizzled3 knock-out mice: a comparison of diffusion tensor magnetic resonance imaging, neurofilament staining, and genetically directed cell labeling. J Neurosci 2006;26:355–364.
69 Bui T, Daire JL, Chalard F, Zaccaria I, Alberti C, Elmaleh M, Garel C, Luton D, Blanc N, Sebag G: Microstructural development of human brain assessed in utero by diffusion tensor imaging. Pediatr Radiol 2006;36:1133–1140.
70 Schneider JF, Confort-Gouny S, Le Fur Y, Viout P, Bennathan M, Chapon F, Fogliarini C, Cozzone P, Girard N: Diffusion-weighted imaging in normal fetal brain maturation. Eur Radiol 2007;17:2422–2429.
71 Kroenke CD, Bretthorst GL, Inder TE, Neil JJ: Diffusion MR imaging characteristics of the developing primate brain. Neuroimage 2005;25:1205–1213.
72 Duhaime AC, Saykin AJ, McDonald BC, Dodge CP, Eskey CJ, Darcey TM, Grate LL, Tomashosky P: Functional magnetic resonance imaging of the primary somatosensory cortex in piglets. J Neurosurg 2006;104:259–264.
73 Wai MS, Rudd JA, Chan WY, Antonio GE, Yew DT: The effect of Ginkgo biloba on the cerebellum of aging SAMP mouse – a TUNEL, bcl-2, and fMRI study. Microsc Res Tech 2007;70:671–676.
74 Zhang L, Li Q, Wolff LT, Antonio GE, Yeung DK, Zhang A, Wu Y, Yew DT: Changes of brain activity in the aged SAMP mouse. Biogerontology 2007;8:81–88.
75 Fang M, Lorke DE, Li J, Gong X, Yew JC, Yew DT: Postnatal changes in functional activities of the pig's brain: a combined functional magnetic resonance imaging and immunohistochemical study. Neurosignals 2005;14:222–233.
76 Fang M, Zhang L, Li J, Wang C, Chung CH, Wai SM, Yew DT: The postnatal development of the cerebellum – a fMRI and silver study. Cell Mol Neurobiol 2005;25:1043–1050.
77 Fang M, Li J, Rudd JA, Wai SM, Yew JC, Yew DT: fMRI mapping of cortical centers following visual stimulation in postnatal pigs of different ages. Life Sci 2006;78:1197–1201.
78 Gothelf D, Hoeft F, Hinard C, Hallmayer JF, Stoecker JV, Antonarakis SE, Morris MA, Reiss AL: Abnormal cortical activation during response inhibition in 22q11.2 deletion syndrome. Hum Brain Mapp 2007;28:533–542.
79 Smith LM, Chang L, Yonekura ML, Gilbride K, Kuo J, Poland RE, Walot I, Ernst T: Brain proton magnetic resonance spectroscopy and imaging in children exposed to cocaine in utero. Pediatrics 2001;107:227–231.

Neuroembryology and Aging

Neuroembryol Aging 2008;5:49–55
DOI: 10.1159/000116732

Received: November 7, 2007
Accepted: November 22, 2007
Published online: August 19, 2008

Magnetic Resonance Imaging of Fetal Brain Abnormalities

Guowei Tao[a] David T. Yew[b]

[a]Department of Ultrasonography, QiLu Hospital, Shan Dong University, Jinan, and [b]Department of Anatomy, Faculty of Medicine, Chinese University of Hong Kong, Hong Kong, SAR, China

Key Words
Abnormality · Clinical decision-making · Fetal brain · MRI · Neuroimaging · Prenatal sonography

Abstract
Magnetic resonance imaging (MRI) of the fetal brain is a useful adjunct to prenatal sonography, providing a more complete evaluation of fetal brain abnormalities to aid and influence clinical decision-making during pregnancy. This article will review the uses and techniques of fetal MRI, discuss the normal appearance of the fetal brain on MRI, and outline clinical applications of fetal MR imaging.

Introduction

Magnetic resonance imaging (MRI) is an increasingly available technique used to evaluate the fetal brain. Advances in ultrafast scan sequence and coil design have contributed to the clinical use of fetal MRI in determining brain morphology. Fetal MRI has higher contrast resolution than prenatal sonography and excellent soft tissue contrast; it provides multiple planes for reconstruction and a large field of view, allowing for better depiction of the anatomy of fetuses with central nervous system (CNS) abnormalities [1–3]. The objective of this article is to review the state of fetal brain MRI and its application in prenatal diagnosis.

Utility and Limitations of Fetal Brain MRI

In general, ultrasonography is the primary screening modality for obstetric imaging and is usually capable of making the correct diagnoses for many fetal CNS abnormalities. However, sonographic diagnosis is limited by the nonspecific appearance of some anomalies, by limited resolution of the side of the brain nearest the transducer, and by ossification that obscures visualization of posterior fossa structures [4, 5]. Fetal MRI enables direct visualization of the developing brain parenchyma and is not susceptible to the same limitations as ultrasound, thereby allowing better differentiation of normal from abnormal tissue. Major roles for fetal brain MRI include the confirmation of sonographically detected abnormalities and the discovery of additional abnormalities that are otherwise not apparent by sonography [3–5]. With recent advances in fetal surgical techniques, fetal MRI is increasingly used before surgical intervention, for example in Chiari II malformation [6]. Advanced MRI techniques, such as diffusion-weighted imaging (DWI), diffusion tensor imaging (DTI) and proton MR spectroscopy (MRS), have recently also been applied to evaluate fetal brain development and destructive processes [7–10].

At this time, fetal MRI has no known risks to the fetus at the gestational ages of those imaged. Limitations of fetal MRI are mainly related to the artifact of fetal motion. Even with rapid image acquisition, fetal motion can still affect the quality of the images, especially in the first and

KARGER

Fax +41 61 306 12 34
E-Mail karger@karger.ch
www.karger.com

1661–3406/08/0052–0049$24.50/0

Accessible online at:
www.karger.com/nba

Dr. David T. Yew
Department of Anatomy
Chinese University of Hong Kong
Shatin, N.T., Hong Kong, SAR (China)
Tel. +852 2609 6899, Fax +852 2603 5031, E-Mail david-yew@cuhk.edu.hk

second trimester. Another limitation is the small size of the brain structure being imaged, although this issue is being overcome with advances in MR techniques [2, 8]. The customary MRI safety checks apply to the mother regarding metal implants and aneurysm clips, for example [11]. In addition, some pregnant women may have claustrophobia and not be able to tolerate the present requirements of the examination.

MRI Techniques

Fetal MRI is routinely performed on 1.5-tesla scanners. An eight-channel torso phased-array coil is used to allow increased coverage of the fetal head and an increased signal-to-noise ratio compared to more standard pelvic phased-array coils. Ultrafast sequences known as single-shot fast spin echo or half-Fourier acquired single-shot turbo spin-echo are usually used to decrease sensitivity to fetal motion. The T_2-weighted images depict fetal brain anatomy very accurately at different gestational ages and are considered the best sequence for imaging fetal brain abnormalities. The application of T_1-weighted fetal MRI is more limited because of the longer scan time with lower signal-to-noise ratio. At present, fast low-angle shot sequences are the most robust in T_1-weighted imaging. Fat and hemorrhage may be clearly visualized using T_1-weighted images [8, 12].

Advanced MRI techniques for improved visualization of fetal brain tissue include DWI, DTI, proton MRS (^{1}H-MRS) and functional MRI (fMRI). DWI reflects the Brownian motion of water molecules within the brain that can be used to detect early stages of destruction in brain areas. DTI provides information on the direction of the white matter tracts. However, with longer scan time and image susceptibility to fetal and maternal motion, DWI and DTI are still limited in their clinical applications [7, 13]. ^{1}H-MRS is a noninvasive tool for examining cerebral metabolism but is also difficult to perform on the fetus because of its long scan time requirements (about 30 min) without fetal or maternal motion. It is currently used in research protocols. fMRI is based on the blood oxygen level-dependent effect and studies brain activity in response to various stimuli. At present, fMRI applications are also within the realm of research [7, 14].

In conclusion, conventional fetal MRI remains essential for studying fetal brain pathology and morphology. More advanced MRI techniques will likely develop in the near future so that more definitive information about the fetal brain can be gained.

Normal Fetal Brain Appearance on MRI

Interpretation of fetal MR images requires an extensive understanding of embryology. Fetal brain development is characterized by the processes of neuronal migration, gyration and myelination. Cells migrate from the germinal ventricular zone (also called germinal matrix) at 7–8 weeks of gestation. The germinal zone appears hyperintense on T_1-weighted images and markedly hypointense on T_2-weighted images. By week 20, the cortical plate is formed. The cortical plate is highly cellular with packed cells and appears on MRI as a rather bright signal on T_1-weighted images and as a smooth ribbon of low signal on T_2-weighted images. The subplate, a transient structure of the developing human brain, serves as a partner to receive subcortical fiber systems (thalamus, brainstem and basal forebrain) and can be visualized adjacent to the cortical plate. It is widest around the 22nd gestational week (GW) and gradually dissolves after the 30th GW. The subplate appears hypointense on T_1-weighted images and hyperintense on T_2-weighted images compared to the cortical plate. The intermediate zone, a middle region between the germinal ventricular zone and the cortical plate, corresponds to a less cellular region of developing white matter and shows intermediate signal intensity [10, 15–17]. These signals may be explained by the high content of extracellular matrix in the cells and by the variety of synapses composed of aligned ultrastructural elements.

Another aspect of brain development visualized by fetal MRI is the formation of sulci or sulcation. The appearance of the fetal brain changes dramatically from 20 to 35 GW, progressing from an initially smooth and agyric brain to highly complex and convoluted patterns of sulci. Sulcation is a significant indicator of cortical development and maturity, and progresses in a prescribed pattern of specific primary sulci, followed by secondary and tertiary sulci. Primary sulci appear between the 18th and 24th GW, secondary sulci appear around the 24th GW and tertiary sulci appear between the 28th and 37th GW. It is important to note that sulcation of the developing brain on fetal MRI lags slightly behind fetal autopsy specimens, likely due to the greater detail afforded by pathological examinations. Gyration appears later than sulcation in the fetal brain and proceeds cephalad in an orderly fashion, similar to the pattern of myelination [15–18].

Myelination of the brain begins at approximately 20 GW and continues after birth until mature at about 3 years. CNS myelination progresses in predictable sequences from caudal (spinal cord and brainstem) to rostral (telencephalon). In the cortex, myelination spreads in a concentric fashion, whereas myelination in the white matter follows functionally defined bundles, e.g. from sensory tracts to motor tracts. The deposition of myelin can significantly shorten the time of T_1 and T_2 relaxation times, therefore the T_1 hyperintensity and T_2 hypointensity are well observed in the fetal MRI as myelination progresses [16, 17, 19].

Classification of Congenital Anomalies in the CNS

Van der Knaap and Valk [20] proposed a classification system of congenital abnormalities of the CNS based on MRI appearance and organized in terms of the timing of gestational disturbances. During the major 'formational' period, for example up to 5–7 GW, insults result in primary malformations of the CNS. These malformations include: disorders of dorsal and ventral neural tube formation; disorders of neuronal, glial and mesenchymal proliferation, differentiation and histogenesis, and disorders of migration and cortical organization. Conditions may include encephaloceles, Chiari malformations, holoprosencephaly, Dandy-Walker malformation, schizencephaly, gray matter heterotopias or dysgenesis of the corpus callosum, for example. Insults that occur during the post-formational period of maturation, for example after 5–7 GW, result in 'secondary' injuries of formed structures. Such injuries may include hydranencephaly, porencephaly, multicystic encephalopathy, hemorrhage, encephalomalacia and infarction.

For some serious malformations (i.e. anencephalus, meningocele, hydrocephalus or classic Dandy-Walker malformation), sonography can make an accurate diagnosis, but prenatal sonography is limited in its ability to detect many of the destructive developmental lesions, such as agenesis of the corpus callosum, sulcation anomalies, periventricular nodular heterotopia, hemorrhage and cerebella dysplasia [5, 21–24]. Fetal MRI can detect sonographically occult abnormalities for a variety of indications in up to 50% of the cases studied [12, 25].

In this next section, we will review the most common and important congenital abnormalities of the CNS using fetal MRI according to the classification of van der Knaap and Valk [20].

Clinical Applications of Fetal MRI

Disorders of Ventral Neural Tube Development

Holoprosencephaly

Ventral neural tube development refers to the inductive events occurring in the rostral end of the embryo, resulting in the formation of the face and brain at 5–10 GW [26]. The prosencephalon divides into the telencephalon and diencephalon during normal brain development. Holoprosencephaly is a spectrum of malformations of the prosencephalon, including three main types in decreasing severity: alobar, semilobar and lobar holoprosencephaly. Alobar holoprosencephaly is attributed to a lack of differentiation resulting in a single prosencephalic vesicle, with a single ventricular cavity instead of the third and lateral ventricles, and no septum pellucidum. The falx cerebri, interhemispheric fissure and corpus callosum are absent. Other brain abnormalities include fusion of the globes, absent or abnormal olfactory bulbs, and an atrophic or hypoplastic pituitary gland. Obviously, these abnormalities may be more or less severe, depending on the possible etiologic processes. The most severe forms of facial dysmorphia are generally associated with this type. Semilobar holoprosencephaly shows the interhemispheric fissure and falx cerebri are partly present at the back of the brain. Fusion and lack of brain development are observed. The thalami are partly fused. Lobar holoprosencephaly, the least severe form, shows the presence of the falx cerebri at the front (more or less poorly developed), yet the third ventricle is completely formed. The frontal horns are partially developed and the temporal horns are neatly individualized. The callosal fibers of the corpus callosum body and the splenium are present [20, 26, 27].

MRI is used to confirm the sonographic diagnosis and distinguish the type of holoprosencephaly. Moreover, if maternal body habitus or reverberation artifacts on the calvaria make it difficult to visualize the falx and other midline structures with ultrasound, then MRI is more conclusive [27–29].

Dandy-Walker Continuum

The cerebellum develops from the alar plate in the dorsal region of the neural tube. Cerebellar primordia begin as symmetrical bulges from laminae on each side of the metencephalic midline at the end of the 6th GW. These lateral elements develop toward the midline and fuse to form the superior and then the inferior vermis [30]. The more lateral elements develop into cerebellar hemispheres.

Numerous theories have been proposed to explain the Dandy-Walker continuum but it remains poorly understood. Its heterogeneity probably explains why this malformation remains difficult to define and classify more than 80 years after its initial description. The Dandy-Walker continuum is commonly composed of three forms: classic Dandy-Walker malformation, the Dandy-Walker variant and mega cisterna magna [31]. Some studies suggest the Blake's pouch cyst should be included in the Dandy-Walker malformation because of the similarities in its condition to the Dandy-Walker syndrome [32]. Dandy-Walker can be sporadic and isolated, or accompanied with other neurological malformations or chromosomal aberrations [31].

Fetal brain MRI is particularly useful in the diagnosis of the Dandy-Walker continuum when sonography is abnormal or doubtful in the second and third trimester. The classic Dandy-Walker malformation includes complete or partial vermian agenesis, cystic dilation of the posterior fossa communicating with the fourth ventricle, and an abnormally high tentorium. The Dandy-Walker variant represents a lesser degree of cerebellar vermis hypogenesis with less dilatation of the fourth ventricle, and less enlargement of the posterior fossa. The mega cisterna magna show the vermis is complete with a separate fourth ventricle, but with a large posterior fossa usually exceeding 10 mm. Blake's pouch cyst represents persistent dorsal expansion of the fourth ventricle. If Blake's pouch is enlarged, it will develop behind and around the cerebellum, pushing the developing tentorium into an abnormally high position [32].

Fetal MRI can be helpful in determining the shape and size of the vermis on different planes in order to differentiate between Dandy-Walker variant and a mega cisterna magna. The position of the tentorium cerebelli and the relationship of the posterior fossa and the fourth ventricle can be clearly seen on sagittal or axial slices [30–34]. When a Dandy-Walker malformation is identified, fetal MRI can be used to detect additional CNS abnormalities, which may include agenesis of the corpus callosum, polymicrogyria, neuronal heterotopia and hydrocephalus. These associated malformations increase the risk of poor neurological outcome. Fetal MRI is particularly valuable in identifying these anomalies [33, 34].

Disorders of Proliferation, Migration and Cortical Organization

Cortical development and maturation are characterized by proliferation, migration and differentiation of CNS cells, especially neurons. Cellular proliferation starts by 5 GW and takes place from 8 to 16 GW within the germinal ventricular zone [15, 16]. Migration of neuronal and glial stem cells from their site of origin in the periventricular germinal matrix to the cortical and subcortical areas of the brain occurs primarily from 3 to 5 months of gestation. Two types of neuronal migration are described by histology: radial and tangential migration. Radial migration involves the future pyramidal neurons migrating from the germinal ventricular zone along the radial glial fibers in an inside-out fashion. The first neurons to migrate form the deep layers of the cortex and the late migrating cells form the superficial layers of the cortex. Tangential migration represents 12% of neuronal migration, involves the interneurons that migrate from the ganglionic eminences and uses astrocytes as a support for migration. Following proliferation and migration, the next step of synaptogenesis includes cortical organization and cellular differentiation. Synaptogenesis is characterized by the establishment of networks, with a dramatic increase in cortex and brain weight. Increase in brain volume and weight, and the changes in surface configuration, are mainly due to the developing sulcation [15–16, 35].

Anomalies resulting from disturbed neuronal proliferation, migration and cortical organization mainly include microcephaly, lissencephaly, heterotopia, polymicrogyria, schizencephaly and hypogenesis of the corpus callosum. MRI is better suited than sonography for the prenatal diagnosis of cortical development abnormalities and is able to diagnose 80% of lissencephalies, 73% of polymicrogyrias, 100% of schizencephalies and 54% of neuronal heterotopias [36].

Microcephaly

Microcephaly describes a small head and brain, is defined as a cranial diameter below the 3rd percentile [37] and may constitute another form of brain malformation (holoprosencephaly or schizencephaly). Microlissencephaly is a primitive form of microcephaly with simplified gyral patterns. It may result from a disturbance in the proliferation of neuroblasts in the germinal zone, or from an excess of programmed cellular death, possibly leading to a decrease in the number of glial units and cortical neurons, with an accompanying decrease in the volume of white matter [37, 38].

Fetal MRI plays an essential role in the diagnosis of this malformation. Receding forehead and abnormally small fronto-occipital and biparietal diameters are usually detected. The simplified gyral pattern is clear because only the primary sulci are present, and are abnormally wide and shallow. Secondary sulci are absent when they are usually detected at 34 GW. Therefore, follow-up is often necessary to confirm no progress in gyration after 34 weeks [38–40].

Lissencephaly

Most lissencephalic brains present a combination of agyria and pachygyria. Agyria is defined as the complete absence of sulci; it is a synonym of complete lissencephaly. Pachygyria is defined as a low number of shallow sulci with an abnormally thick cortex, also termed lissencephaly [29, 38, 41].

Type I lissencephaly (classic lissencephaly) is characterized by a thickened cortex with broad flat gyri, a few shallow sulci and diminished white matter. The brain is described as figure eight shaped due to bilateral opercular dysplasia. The potentially associated abnormalities of the corpus callosum, brain stem and cerebellum are well visualized using MRI [41–43].

Type II lissencephaly (cobblestone lissencephaly) is the more common form of lissencephaly. The cortex has a chaotic aspect, the layers are not clearly individualized and the neurons appear disoriented. Type II lissencephaly appears in some syndromes, with Walker-Warburg syndrome being the most frequently observed in antenatal MRI. Its main signs are ventricular dilatation, abnormalities in the posterior fossa and ocular abnormalities. Associated anomalies include subcortical heterotopias, callosal hypogenesis, cerebellar cortical dysplasia and cerebellar vermian hypoplasia [41, 42, 44].

Polymicrogyria

Polymicrogyria is characterized by the presence of numerous small gyri with intervening sulci. As a consequence, the brain surface appears abnormally smooth with some irregular sulci. On MRI, polymicrogyria appears as a slightly thickened and irregular cortex with shallow sulci. Fetal MRI shows the features of polymicrogyria better than ultrasound, but it is likely that most cases are missed by routine US examination. There are therefore limited MRI records of this condition in the fetal state [28, 45–47].

Schizencephaly

Schizencephaly is characterized by a cerebrospinal fluid (CSF)-filled cleft lined with gray matter between the lateral ventricle and the surface of the cortex. The cleft may be closed (fused lips) or open (open lips) by a cavity that may or may not communicate with the ventricle. The cleft is commonly located in the perisylvian region and can be uni- or bilateral, symmetrical or asymmetrical. The associated disorders include polymicrogyria, heterotopia, callosal hypogenesis and absence of the septum pellucidum [28, 48].

MRI offers a clear view of the cortex lining the cleft; abnormal sulci are often noted, indicating polymicrogyria and gray matter heterotopia lining the cleft. Also, distinguishing open-lip schizencephaly from porencephaly and arachnoid cysts is more accurate with MRI than US [37, 38].

Neuronal Heterotopia

Neuronal heterotopias are collections of neurons in abnormal locations that may occur in subependymal, subcortical or intracortical sites [49].

Subependymal heterotopia appears as nodules that are isointense to the germinal matrix and are located along the ventricular walls. An irregularity in the ventricular wall is an essential sign of heterotopia. These heterotopias can be focal or diffuse, uni- or bilateral. They may be isolated or associated with other malformations such as corpus callosum agenesis. They cannot be reliably distinguished from subependymal nodules as seen in tuberous sclerosis, therefore it is important to search for additional manifestations of tuberous sclerosis [28, 37, 50].

Subcortical heterotopia is less frequent than subependymal heterotopia. They are often sporadic and difficult to detect on prenatal MRI when they are dispersed throughout the white matter. Dysgenesis of the corpus callosum is found in 70% of cases [38]. Intracortical heterotopia may appear when neuronal migration ceases in the deepest layers of the cortex [37].

Hypogenesis of the Corpus Callosum

At 11–12 GW, the corpus callosum begins to develop dorsal to the hippocampal commissure, growing caudally along with the cerebral hemispheres. By 18 GW, all the components of the corpus callosum should be present [29, 50]. Because of its relatively late development, various brain anomalies are often associated with abnormalities in the corpus callosum. Brain abnormalities seen in association with callosal agenesis include Arnold-Chiari II malformation, Dandy-Walker malformation, gray matter heterotopia, holoprosencephaly, schizencephaly and encephaloceles. The prognosis of hypogenesis of the corpus callosum is poor when associated with other abnormalities in the CNS [29, 37, 51].

Hypogenesis of the corpus callosum can be partial or complete, as the interhemispheric cerebral axonal fibers may not fully migrate across the midline. The residual commissural fibers are distributed longitudinally as Probst bundles [51]. Indirect signs of hypogenesis of the corpus callosum include lack of visualization of the cavum septi pellucidi, with enlarged atria and occipital horns of the lateral ventricles in a teardrop configuration, a high-riding third ventricle and radiating medial hemispheric sulci [24, 52].

A direct sonographic visualization of the entire corpus callosum on a midline sagittal image is difficult to obtain. Fetal MRI has greater sensitivity compared to prenatal sonography in the detection of callosal hypogenesis, callosal agenesis and associated brain anomalies. In contrast to the indirect appearance of ultrasound, MRI can demonstrate clear and direct visualization in the sagittal and coronal planes [24, 25].

Encephaloclastic Abnormalities of the Developing CNS

Encephaloclastic abnormalities of the fetal brain include congenital infections, hemorrhage, hydranencephaly, porencephaly, encephalomalacia and hydrocephalus [20].

Infections and Hemorrhage

Congenital viral infection is a frequent indication for fetal MRI, affording more accurate identification of abnormalities of the affected developing brain parenchyma and cortex. The most common cause of congenital viral infection is cytomegalovirus. Areas of chronic parenchymal injury typically appear bright on T_2-weighted images and can be focal or diffuse. Chronic injury may also be manifested by volume loss and ventricular enlargement [53, 54].

Hemorrhage is usually visualized as areas of hypointensity on T_2-weighted images or hyperintensity on T_1-weighted images, although the signal intensity can vary depending on the stage of hemorrhage. Hemorrhage can occur within the ventricle, appearing as layers of debris in the dependent portion of the ventricle, or as a focal hematoma, or within the adjacent brain parenchyma. The detection of small subependymal hemorrhages is more difficult. T_2-weighted gradient-echo sequences may be used to confirm the presence of blood due to hemorrhage appearing more hypointense than the germinal matrix [53, 55].

Porencephaly

Porencephaly may result from necrosis caused by infection, trauma, hemorrhage or infarction and is defined as a CSF-containing cavity that may or may not communicate with the ventricles or the subarachnoid space. In fetal MRI, porencephaly has the same signal intensity as CSF on T_1-weighted and T_2-weighted images; however, it is unilateral or asymmetrical in most cases. The differential diagnosis includes arachnoid cyst and cystic tumors. Arachnoid cysts are always in a basal, anterior temporal or interhemispheric location; cystic tumors usually grow rapidly and may have a mass effect [38, 55].

Conclusion

In conclusion, fetal brain MRI has become an increasingly useful and important adjunct to prenatal sonography, particularly for definitive evaluation of fetal brain abnormalities. Imaging advancements and improved accuracy provide more and better information regarding abnormalities of the fetal brain, which will allow better-informed clinical decisions during pregnancy.

References

1 Levine D, Barnes PD, Edelman RR: Obstetric MR imaging. Radiology 1999;211:609–617.

2 Girard N, Raybaud C, Gambarelli D, Figarella-Branger D: Fetal brain MR imaging. Magn Reson Imaging Clin N Am 2001;9:19–56.

3 Merzoug V, Ferey S, Andre Ch, Gelot A, Adamsbaum C: Magnetic resonance imaging of the fetal brain. J Neuroradiol 2002;29:76–90.

4 Barnewolt CE, Estroff JA: Sonography of the fetal central nervous system. Neuroimaging Clin N Am 2004;14:255–271.

5 Frates MC, Kumar AJ, Benson CB, Ward VL, Tempany CM: Fetal anomalies: comparison of MR imaging and US for diagnosis. Radiology 2004;232:398–404.

6 Coakley FV: Role of magnetic resonance imaging in fetal surgery. Top Magn Reson Imaging 2001;12:39–51.

7 Garel C: New advances in fetal MR neuroimaging. Pediatr Radiol 2006;36:621–625.

8 Glenn OA, Barkovich AJ: Magnetic resonance imaging of the fetal brain and spine: an increasingly important tool in prenatal diagnosis, part 1. AJNR Am J Neuroradiol 2006;27:1604–1611.

9 Brugger PC, Stuhr F, Lindner C, Prayer D: Methods of fetal MR: beyond T2-weighted imaging. Eur J Radiol 2006;57:172–181.
10 Dietrich RB, Cohen I: Fetal MR imaging. Magn Reson Imaging Clin N Am 2006;14: 503–522.
11 Rich P, Jones R, Britton J, Foote S, Thilaganathan B: MRI of the foetal brain. Clin Radiol 2007;62:303–313.
12 Simon EM, Goldstein RB, Coakley FV, Filly RA, Broderick KC, Musci TJ, Barkovich AJ: Fast MR imaging of fetal CNS anomalies in utero. AJNR Am J Neuroradiol 2000;21: 1688–1698.
13 Agid R, Lieberman S, Nadjari M, Gomori JM: Prenatal MR diffusion-weighted imaging in a fetus with hemimegalencephaly. Pediatr Radiol 2006;36:138–140.
14 Heerschap A, Kok RD, van den Berg PP: Antenatal proton MR spectroscopy of the human brain in vivo. Childs Nerv Syst 2003;19: 418–421.
15 Prayer D, Kasprian G, Krampl E, Ulm B, Witzani L, Prayer L, Brugger PC: MRI of normal fetal brain development. Eur J Radiol 2006;57:199–216.
16 Rados M, Judas M, Kostovic I: In vitro MRI of brain development. Eur J Radiol 2006;57: 187–198.
17 Glenn OA: Fetal central nervous system MR imaging. Neuroimaging Clin N Am 2006;16: 1–17.
18 Abe S, Takagi K, Yamamoto T, Kato T: Assessment of cortical gyrus and sulcus formation using magnetic resonance images in small-for-gestational-age fetuses. Prenat Diagn 2004;24:333–338.
19 Girard N, Raybaud C, Poncet M: In vivo MR study of brain maturation in normal fetuses. AJNR Am J Neuroradiol 1995;16:407–413.
20 van der Knaap MS, Valk J: Classification of congenital abnormalities of the CNS. AJNR Am J Neuroradiol 1988;9:315–326.
21 Malinger G, Lev D, Lerman-Sagie T: Fetal central nervous system: MR imaging versus dedicated US – need for prospective, blind, comparative studies. Radiology 2004;232: 306.
22 Brugger PC, Prayer D: Fetal MRI of pathological brain development. Radiology 2006; 46:112–119.
23 Prayer D: Fetal MR. Eur J Radiol 2006;57: 171.
24 Glenn OA, Barkovich J: Magnetic resonance imaging of the fetal brain and spine: an increasingly important tool in prenatal diagnosis: part 2. AJNR Am J Neuroradiol 2006; 27:1807–1814.
25 Frates MC, Kumar AJ, Benson CB, Ward VL, Tempany CM: Fetal anomalies: comparison of MR imaging and US for diagnosis. Radiology 2004;232:398–404.
26 Joo GJ, Beke A, Papp C, Toth-Pal E, Szigeti Z, Ban Z, Papp Z: Prenatal diagnosis, phenotypic and obstetric characteristics of holoprosencephaly. Fetal Diagn Ther 2005;20: 161–166.
27 Toma P, Costa A, Magnano GM, Cariati M, Lituania M: Holoprosencephaly: prenatal diagnosis by sonography and magnetic resonance imaging. Prenat Diagn 1990;10:429–436.
28 Sonigo PC, Rypens FF, Carteret M, Delezoide AL, Brunelle FO: MR imaging of fetal cerebral anomalies. Pediatr Radiol 1998;28: 212–222.
29 Levine D, Barnes PD: Cortical maturation in normal and abnormal fetuses as assessed with prenatal MR imaging. Radiology 1999; 210:751–758.
30 Stazzone MM, Hubbard AM, Bilaniuk LT, Harty MP, Meyer JS, Zimmerman RA, Mahboubi S: Ultrafast MR imaging of the normal posterior fossa in fetuses. AJR Am J Roentgenol 2000;175:835–839.
31 Glenn OA: Fetal central nervous system MR imaging. Neuroimaging Clin N Am 2006;16: 1–17.
32 Calabrò F, Arcuri T, Jinkins JR: Blake's pouch cyst: an entity within the Dandy-Walker continuum. Neuroradiology 2000; 42:290–295.
33 Chen SC, Simon EM, Haselgrove JC, Bilaniuk LT, Sutton LN, Johnson MP, Shera DM, Zimmerman RA: Fetal posterior fossa volume: assessment with MR imaging. Radiology 2006;238:997–1003.
34 Levine D, Barnes PD, Robertson RR, Wong G, Mehta TS: Fast MR imaging of fetal central nervous system abnormalities. Radiology 2003;229:51–61.
35 Fogliarini C, Chaumoitre K, Chapon F, Fernandez C, Levrier O, Figarella-Branger D, Girard N: Assessment of cortical maturation with prenatal MRI. Part I. Normal cortical maturation. Eur Radiol 2005;15:1671–1685.
36 Sonigo PC, Rypens FF, Carteret M, Delezoide AL, Brunelle FO: MR imaging of fetal cerebral anomalies. Pediatr Radiol 1998;28: 212–222.
37 Garel C: MRI of the Fetal Brain, ed 1. Berlin, Springer, 2004, p 152.
38 Raybaud C, Levrier O, Brunel H, Girard N, Farnarier P: MR imaging of fetal brain malformations. Childs Nerv Syst 2003;19:455–470.
39 Steinlin M, Zurrer M, Martin E, Boesch C, Largo RH, Boltshauser E: Contribution of magnetic resonance imaging in the evaluation of microcephaly. Neuropediatrics 1991; 22:184–189.
40 Peiffer A, Singh N, Leppert M, Dobyns WB, Carey JC: Microcephaly with simplified gyral pattern in six related children. Am J Med Genet 1999;84:137–144.
41 Ghai S, Fong KW, Toi A, Chitayat D, Pantazi S, Blaser S: Prenatal US and MR imaging findings of lissencephaly: review of fetal cerebral sulcal development. Radiographics 2006;26:389–405.
42 Lee BC, Engel M: MR of lissencephaly. AJNR Am J Neuroradiol 1988;9:804.
43 de Rijk-van Andel JF, van der Knaap MS, Valk J, Arts WF: Neuroimaging in lissencephaly type I. Neuroradiology 1991;33:230–233.
44 Takanashi J, Tada H, Fujii K, Barkovich AJ: The evolving MR imaging appearance of lissencephaly: a case report. Brain Dev 2007;29: 522–524.
45 Barkovich AJ, Rowley H, Bollen A: Correlation of prenatal events with the development of polymicrogyria. AJNR Am J Neuroradiol 1995;16:822–827.
46 Takanashi J, Barkovich AJ: The changing MR imaging appearance of polymicrogyria: a consequence of myelination. AJNR Am J Neuroradiol 2003;24:788–793.
47 Widjaja E, Wilkinson ID, Griffiths PD: Magnetic resonance perfusion imaging in malformations of cortical development. Acta Radiol 2007;48:907–917.
48 Boardman JP, Dyet LE: Recent advances in imaging preterm brain injury. Minerva Pediatr 2007;59:349–368.
49 Barkovich AJ, Guerrini R, Battaglia G, Kalifa G, N'Guyen T, Parmeggiani A, Santucci M, Giovanardi-Rossi P, Granata T, D'Incerti L: Band heterotopia: correlation of outcome with magnetic resonance imaging parameters. Ann Neurol 1994;36:609–617.
50 Gabrielli O, Carloni I, Coppa GV: MR analysis of the corpus callosum. AJNR Am J Neuroradiol 1997;18:1793–1794.
51 Bekker MN, van Vugt JM: The role of magnetic resonance imaging in prenatal diagnosis of fetal anomalies. Eur J Obstet Gynecol Reprod Biol 2001;96:173–178.
52 Garel C: Fetal cerebral biometry: normal parenchymal findings and ventricular size. Eur Radiol 2005;15:809–813.
53 Girard N, Gire C, Sigaudy S, Porcu G, d'Ercole C, Figarella-Branger D, Raybaud C, Confort-Gouny S: MR imaging of acquired fetal brain disorders. Childs Nerv Syst 2003; 19:490–500.
54 Brunel H, Girard N, Confort-Gouny S, Viola A, Chaumoitre K, D'ercole C, Figarella-Branger D, Raybaud C, Cozzone P, Panuel M: Fetal brain injury. J Neuroradiol 2004;31: 123–137.
55 Prayer D, Brugger PC, Kasprian G, Witzani L, Helmer H, Dietrich W, Eppel W, Langer M: MRI of fetal acquired brain lesions. Eur J Radiol 2006;57:233–249.

Neuroembryology and Aging

Neuroembryol Aging 2008;5:56–59
DOI: 10.1159/000116733

Received: November 19, 2007
Accepted: November 29, 2007
Published online: August 19, 2008

Use of Functional Magnetic Resonance Imaging (Blood Oxygenation Level-Dependent Imaging, Diffusion Tensor Imaging and Magnetic Resonance Spectroscopy) in Brain Development Research

Fei Fei Yang[a] Shu Guang Yuan[a] David T. Yew[b]

[a]Department of Radiology, Second Affiliated Hospital of Kunming Medical College, Kunming, and
[b]Department of Anatomy, Chinese University of Hong Kong, Hong Kong, SAR, China

Key Words
Blood oxygen level-dependent imaging · Brain · Development · Diffusion tensor imaging · Functional magnetic resonance imaging · Magnetic resonance spectroscopy

Abstract
The development of several new magnetic resonance imaging (MRI) techniques has facilitated serial observations of the developing human brain in utero. For example, the noninvasive technique of functional MRI, which is used to study brain anatomy, function and metabolism in both humans and animals, has already enhanced our understanding of brain development and behavior relations. Currently, three main kinds of functional MRI techniques are used to study the developing brain: blood oxygenation level-dependent imaging, diffusion tensor imaging and magnetic resonance spectroscopy. When used in developmental research, these techniques can detect variations and injury, which conventional MRI cannot. Thus, they offer far greater opportunities to explore the relationships between structure and function, and to interpret developmental mechanisms, as well as to detect malformations and pathologies at the cognitive, emotional and behavioral level. These methodologies and their application to brain development are reviewed in this paper.

Introduction

There are several types of functional magnetic resonance imaging (fMRI) techniques. These include: (1) the mapping of cortical function via blood oxygen level-dependent (BOLD) imaging; (2) diffusion-weighted imaging (DWI); (3) diffusion tensor imaging (DTI); (4) magnetic resonance spectroscopy (MRS), and (5) perfusion-weighted imaging. The evolution of these various different noninvasive techniques, which all have good spatial resolution, has revolutionized our progress in neuroimaging research. Three of the techniques, BOLD, DTI and MRS, are increasingly being applied to study different aspects of brain development, e.g. the formation of cortical centers, white matter myelination and connectivity of the brain areas as well as brain metabolism and pathology across the life span.

BOLD

BOLD-based fMRI is a technique used to determine which areas of the brain are active at any particular time. It utilizes the magnetic differences between oxygenated and deoxygenated blood to generate BOLD signals. When neuronal activity occurs, the regional cerebral blood flow (CBF) increases. There is thus a mismatch between the

KARGER

Fax +41 61 306 12 34
E-Mail karger@karger.ch
www.karger.com

1661–3406/08/0052–0056$24.50/0

Accessible online at:
www.karger.com/nba

Dr. David T. Yew
Department of Anatomy
Chinese University of Hong Kong
Shatin, N.T., Hong Kong, SAR (China)
Tel. +852 2609 6899, Fax +852 2603 5031, E-Mail david-yew@cuhk.edu.hk

CBF and the cerebral metabolic rate of oxygen, and this change results in an increase in the capillary and venous oxygenation level (i.e. the level of oxygenated and deoxygenated hemoglobin increases and decreases, respectively). As hemoglobin becomes paramagnetic in the deoxygenated state, this feature makes it a naturally occurring contrast agent, and thus, it can be directly compared with the oxygenated blood. An increase in CBF can therefore be detected as an increase in the MR signal from that particular location of the brain [1, 2]. This change in signal provides the base measure of fMRI and allows for spatial resolution in the order of just a few millimeters [3, 4], with a temporal resolution of as little as a few seconds [5, 6].

BOLD imaging can thus be used to detect subtle changes in the local activity of the brain cortex in response to functional motor, sensory and cognitive tasks. Indeed, it has already been utilized to investigate numerous aspects of brain function, from the most simple motor tasks to complex cognitive functions involving memory-based face recognition, the exploration of language reception and expression, calculating mathematical problems, spatial perception and the changes that occur during psychiatric disorders. It is thought that this technique has the potential to yield significant information regarding the development of language and learning.

BOLD imaging is also being used to study the connectivity of the brain in relationship to the maturational stages of the white matter as well as cortical pruning, brain plasticity and normal brain asymmetry. This technique is being used to determine both where and when maturational changes occur in the brain and how these changes relate to the development of cognitive abilities [7].

There are many anatomical and physiological differences between children and adults. Children undergo many changes in the first years of life. In the first 5 years, for example, the brain increases in volume to 95% of the adult size [8, 9]. Myelination is almost complete by the end of the 2nd year [10, 11]. In addition, the number of brain synapses peaks at around 8 months of age and this is followed by selective synaptic regression in which sprouts are pruned until the age of 16 years [12]. The development of the nervous system occurs via the interaction of several synchronized processes, some of which are complete before birth, while others continue into adulthood [13]. These dynamic structural changes result in a higher metabolism in the younger brain. However, previous research suggests that the BOLD response is quite similar in both children and adolescents, relative to adults. In addition, although there is variability between individuals, to date most of the developmental research has shown fairly similar activation patterns in both children and adults [14–17]. Furthermore, by measuring both the time course and peak amplitude of the BOLD response, recent research has found similar hemodynamic responses in children and adults with similar behavioral performances [18]. On the other hand, Gaillard et al. [15] reported that language tasks in children generate a greater number of activated voxels and frequently bilateral activation compared with adults.

While much of the current information obtained by this technique has been mainly from school-age children and adults, as yet very little is known about newborn brain function. This paucity of data is due to the constraints of the fMRI environment, which requires complete motion restriction. In infants and small children, sedation is often required, and the medications may have a direct effect on CBF and cortical metabolism [19]. However, in cases where sedation has been performed, fMRI has yielded important information regarding the developmental changes that occur in infants and children, such as visual, auditory, language and motor mapping of cortical centers of different ages [19]. Such researches reported that the visual cortex of children >2 years of age show a linear relationship between the number of voxels activated and age. In addition, unilateral damage to the optic radiation produces strong asymmetrical activation [20].

It should also be noted that when BOLD-based fMRI is carried out, appropriate tasks that children can complete are required. The participants (both adults and children) should accommodate to the scanner environment and understand the tasks in advance, especially children.

DTI

While BOLD-based fMRI cannot be used to assess the maturation of projections between brain regions, another fMRI technique, DTI, is currently being used in an effort to trace fiber tracts within the brain [21]. DTI was recently developed from the DWI technique. It relies on the fact that the free movement of water molecules in the human brain is restricted in different directions. The diffusion constant (Dav) is a measure of the amount by which water diffusion is restricted in brain tissue, diffusion anisotropy refers to the ability of water to move in certain directions according to the orientation of the white matter fiber tracts surrounding it and the diffusion tensor is a mathematical description of diffusion [22]. In neonates, Dav should be high and anisotropy should be low, given the increased water content in the brain and the fewer myelinated axons compared with these parameters in adults. As myelination proceeds with development, D_{av} should decrease and anisotropy should increase. By the age of 2 years, myelination is nearly complete and D_{av} and anisotropy values begin to resemble those measured in healthy adults [23–29]. Previous investigators [23, 29] have reported that myelination progresses from inferior to superior, from posterior to anterior, and from central to peripheral (i.e. centrifugal) locations. Thus, DTI can be used in research and applied to the study of white matter fiber tracts to produce diffusion tensor tractography. Several groups have quantified D_{av} and anisotropy, and used these comparative measurements as neuroimaging markers of normal brain maturation in children [24–28]. Thus, alterations in D_{av} and anisotropy in white matter fiber tracts, as quantified using DTI, may be useful sensitive markers of white matter injury or disruption in children with developmental delay. Furthermore, it should be possible to use DTI to reliably quantify changes in myelination as a function of development, and to better assess the effects of maturation in brain structures and brain networks on performance and activation.

MRS

MRS can provide the noninvasive detection of a number of biologically important cellular metabolites. Regional changes in metabolite concentrations during human brain development were assessed by quantitative localized proton MRS in vivo. Significant variations in the concentration of intracellular metabolite levels have been observed in the neonatal brain regarding anatomic location and development. During infancy and childhood, for example, the concentration of the neuroaxonally located N-acetylaspartate acid (NAA) increased in the gray matter, cerebellum and thalamus, whereas a constant level was detected in the white matter. These findings are in line with regional differences identified in the formation of synaptic connections during early development, and suggest a role for NAA as a marker of functioning neuroaxonal tissue rather than of the mere presence of nerve cells [30]. Remarkably, in the basal ganglia, both NAA and taurine remain constant at relatively high concentrations. Other metabolite changes that have been measured by MRS include increases in N-acetylaspartylglutamate, especially in the thalamus and white matter, and a decrease in glutamine in the white matter, all of which occur during maturation [30]. Recently, this technique was applied to provide a unique assessment of the brain biochemistry in the normal neonatal population in order to improve our understanding of brain maturation as well as to establish normative values for the differentiation of abnormal metabolism in cases of brain injury [31]. MRS was also used to demonstrate that normal brain development may be affected in children infected with HIV at birth, particularly evidenced by the lack of the normal age-related increases in NAA concentration [32]. Following this study, recommendations were made for the early, aggressive treatment of infants with HIV before the onset of encephalopathy [32]. In addition, Kreis et al. [33] showed that the absolute metabolite content measured in premature infant brains at term was not considerably different from that in full-term infants. These results indicate that prematurity (but not infants of extremely low birth weight) does not substantially affect the maturation of the normal brain biochemistry [33]. Not only can the biochemical maturation of the brain be studied by MRS in human infants, it can also be investigated in utero in the human fetal brain [34]. A significant reduction in myoinositol and choline, and an increase in NAA concentration were observed with progressive fetal age. Again, this normal MRS data acquired [34] will help to determine whether brain metabolism is altered in cases of in utero injury and disease.

Conclusions

As a relatively new field of research, there are many questions yet to be explored; however, developmental neuroimaging provides an unprecedented opportunity to formulate and test hypotheses that were inaccessible a decade ago. The combination of developmental research and neuroimaging methods has already produced a better understanding of the relationships between cognitive and brain development. Although the various different fMRI techniques provide safe and reliable methods for exploring the brain structures and networks that underlie cognitive abilities, a great deal of care is still needed when acquiring and analyzing the developmental data. Both MRI and fMRI are quite sensitive to artifacts produced by subject motion. Even small movements of the head and neck can significantly reduce the quality of the images. These artifacts can be a particular concern when working with young children. Head restraints (e.g. pillows, foam padding, head and chin straps or bite bars) and periodic reminders are necessary to help participants to lie still and minimize head motion. In addition, it is important to reduce anxiety in order to minimize motion artifacts for both children and adult participants.

References

1 Kwong KK, Belliveau JW, Chesler DA: Dynamic magnetic resonance imaging of human brain activity during primary sensory stimulation. Proc Natl Acad Sci USA 1992; 89:5675–5679.

2 Ogawa S, Lee TS, Nayak AS: Oxygenation-sensitive contrast in magnetic resonance image of rodent brain at high magnetic field. Magn Reson Med 1990;26:68–78.

3 Hu X, Le TH, Ugurbil K: Evaluation of the early response in fMRI in individual subjects using short stimulus duration. Magn Reson Med 1997;37:855–864.

4 Menon RS, Ogawa S, Hu X, Strupp JP, Anderson P, Ugurbil K: BOLD based functional MRI at 4 Tesla includes a capillary bed contribution: echo-planar imaging correlates with previous optical imaging using intrinsic signals. Magn Reson Med 1995;33:453–459.

5 Boynton GM, Engel SA, Glover GH, Heeger DJ: Linear systems analysis of functional magnetic resonance imaging in human V1. J Neurosci 1996;16:4207–4221.

6 Dale AM, Buckner RL: Selective averaging of rapidly presented individual trials using fMRI. Hum Brain Mapp 1997;5:329–340.

7 Casey BJ, Davidson MC, Rosen BR: Functional magnetic resonance imaging: basic principles of and application to developmental science. Dev Sci 2002;5:301–309.

8 Pfefferbaum A, Mathalon DH, Sullivan EV: A quantitative magnetic resonance study of changes in brain morphology from infancy to late adulthood. Arch Neurol 1994;52:874–887.

9 Reiss AL, Abrams MT, Singer HS: Brain development, gender and IQ in children. A volumetric imaging study. Brain 1996;119: 1763–1774.

10 Barkovich AJ, Kjos BO, Jackson D Jr: Normal maturation of the neonatal and infant brain: MR imaging at 1.5 T. Radiology 1988;166: 173–180.

11 Staudt M, Krageloh-Mann I, Grodd W: Normal myelination in childhood brain using MRI – a meta analysis (in German). Rofo 2000;172:802–811.

12 Huttenlocher PR: Synaptic density in human frontal cortex – developmental changes and effects of aging. Brain Res 1979;163:195–205.

13 Lenroot RK, Giedd JN: Brain development in children and adolescents: insights from anatomical magnetic resonance imaging. Neurosci Biobehav Rev 2006;30:718–729.

14 Casey BJ, Cohen JD, Jezzard P, Turner R, Noll DC, Trainor RJ, Giedd J, Kaysen D, Hertz-Pannier L, Rapoport JL: Activation of prefrontal cortex in children during a nonspatial working memory task with functional MRI. Neuroimage 1995;2:221–229.

15 Gaillard WD, Hertz-Pannier L, Mott SH, Barnett AS, LeBihan D, Theodore WH: Functional anatomy of cognitive development: fMRI of verbal fluency in children and adults. Neurology 2000;54:180–185.

16 Nelson CA, Monk CS, Lin J: Functional neuroanatomy of spatial working memory in children. Dev Psychol 2000;36:109–116.

17 Thomas KM, King SW, Frazen PL, Welsh TF, Berkowitz AL, Noll DC, Birmaher V, Casey BJ: A developmental functional MRI study of spatial working memory. Neuroimage 1999; 10:327–338.

18 Schlagger BL, Brown TT, Lugar HM, Visscher KM, Miezin FM, Petersen SE: Functional neuroanatomical differences between adults and school age children in the processing of single words. Science 2002;296:1476–1479.

19 Altman NR, Bernal B: Pediatric applications of fMRI; in Faro SH, Mohamed FB (eds): Functional MRI: Basic Principles and Clinical Applications. New York, Springer, 2006, pp 394–428.

20 Born AP, Miranda MJ, Rostrup E: Functional magnetic resonance imaging of the normal and abnormal visual system in early life. Neuropediatrics 2000;31:24–32.

21 Watts R, Liston C, Niogi S: Fiber tracking using magnetic resonance diffusion tensor imaging and its applications to human brain development. Ment Retard Dev Disabil Res Rev 2003;9:168–177.

22 Rivkin MJ: Developmental neuroimaging of children using magnetic resonance techniques. Ment Retard Dev Disabil Res Rev 2000;6:68–80.

23 Barkovich AJ: Concepts of myelin and myelination in neuroradiology. AJNR Am J Neuroradiol 2000;21:1099–1109.

24 Nomura Y, Sakuma H, Takeda K, Tagami T, Okuda Y, Nakagawa T: Diffusional anisotropy of the human brain assessed with diffusion-weighted MR: relation with normal brain development and aging. AJNR Am J Neuroradiol 1994;15:231–238.

25 Sakuma H, Nomura A, Takeda K: Adult and neonatal human brain: diffusional anisotropy and myelination with diffusion-weighted MR imaging. Radiology 1991;180:229–233.

26 Morriss MC, Zimmerman RA, Bilaniuk LT, Hunter JV, Haselgrove JC: Changes in brain water diffusion during childhood. Neuroradiology 1999;41:929–934.

27 Sakuma H, Nomura Y, Takeda K, Tagami T, Okuda Y, Nakagawa T: Diffusion anisotropy of the human brain assessed with diffusion-weighted MR: relation with normal brain development and aging. AJNR Am J Neuroradiol 1994;15:231–238.

28 Neil JJ, Shiran SI, McKinstry RC, Schefft GL, Snyder AZ, Almli CR, Akbudak E, Aronovitz JA, Miller JP, Lee BC, Conturo TE: Normal brain in human newborns: apparent diffusion coefficient and diffusion anisotropy measured by using diffusion tensor MR imaging. Radiology 1998;209:57–66.

29 Huppi PS, Maier SE, Peled S, Zientara GP, Barnes PD, Jolesz FA, Volpe JJ: Microstructural development of human newborn cerebral white matter assessed in vivo by diffusion tensor magnetic resonance imaging. Pediatr Res 1998;44:584–590.

30 Pouwels PJ, Brockmann K, Kruse B, Wilken B, Wick M, Hanefeld F, Frahm J: Regional age dependence of human brain metabolites from infancy to adulthood as detected by quantitative localized proton MRS. Pediatr Res 1999;46:474–485.

31 Vigneron DB: Magnetic resonance spectroscopic imaging of human brain development. Neuroimaging Clin N Am 2006;16: 75–85.

32 Keller MA, Venkatraman TN, Thomas A, Deveikis A, LoPresti C, Hayes J, Berman N, Walot I, Padilla S, Johnston Jones J, Ernst T, Chang L: Altered neurometabolite development in HIV-infected children: correlation with neuropsychological tests. Neurology 2004;62:1810–1817.

33 Kreis R, Hofmann L, Kuhlmann B, Boesch C, Bossi E, Huppi PS: Brain metabolite composition during early human brain development as measured by quantitative in vivo 1H magnetic resonance spectroscopy. Magn Reson Med 2002;48:949–958.

34 Girard N, Fogliarini C, Viola A, Confort Gouny S, Fur YL, Viout P, Chapon F, Levrier O, Cozzone P: MRS of normal and impaired fetal brain development. Eur J Radiol 2006; 57:217–225.

Neuroembryology and Aging

Neuroembryol Aging 2008;5:60–62
DOI: 10.1159/000116734

Received: October 17, 2007
Accepted: November 2, 2007
Published online: August 19, 2008

Morphometric Measurements of Fetal and Neonatal Eyes Using MRI and Ultrasound

Xi Ying[a] Hai-tao Li[b] David T. Yew[c]

Departments of [a]Ophthalmology and [b]Radiology, Southwest Hospital, Third Military Medical University, Chongqing, and [c]Department of Anatomy, Chinese University of Hong Kong, Hong Kong, SAR, China

Key Words
AP diameter · Transverse diameter · Eye growth · Fetus · Child

Abstract
Using MRI, the ratios of the anterior posterior (AP) lengths of the eyes versus the AP lengths of the corneae to the external occipital protuberances were found to decrease from 28 weeks of gestation onwards, while the ratios of the transverse diameters of the eyes versus the transverse diameters of the zygomatic bone to the nasal cavity increased till term. No further change in the ratios of the AP or transverse diameters was observed even till three years of age.

The growth of the orbit and in particular the growth of the eyeball is an important topic in the evaluation of myopia before school starts. While much research has been conducted in the ocular parameters in school children, research on ocular development in prenatal and neonatal eyes appeared rarely in studies [1–6]. In a radiographic study of 30 fetuses at 18–41 weeks of gestation [1], the corneal, orbital and the biparietal diameters were measured. The results from that study showed a good correlation between the ocular and the biparietal diameters. In another study in the same group [2], the axial lengths of the same fetuses (18–41 weeks of gestation) were assessed by ultrasound and it was concluded that head circumferences correlated best with ocular growth. Goldstein et al. [4], using ultrasound and working with fetuses at 14–36 weeks of gestation, reported on the other hand, (1) a linear growth function between orbital circumference and biparietal diameter and (2) a linear growth function between gestational age and the diameter of the lens.

In the last decade, few studies assessed fetal and neonatal relative eye growth in comparison with skull structures. Dilmen et al. [5] reported that there were indeed linear growth functions between biparietal and lens diameters, as well as between biparietal and orbital diameters in fetuses at 15–40 weeks of gestation. Tomasik et al. [6], working with fetuses at 17–28 weeks of gestation, concluded that axial lengths, equational diameters, depths and widths of the orbit all increased with age: growth of axial length was parallel to the increase in the equational diameter while growth of the equational diameter coincided with the increase in orbital width.

Morphometric studies of this sort have been useful in understanding the growth of the eye in the fetal period. There are, however, several shortcomings. Firstly, there were apparently very few studies in the neonatal period. Secondly, although in some studies one measurement correlated with another measurement, e.g. orbital with equational diameter, these two measurements were often not made along the same line, and radiographic or sonographic planes were not entirely horizontal or transverse and were sometimes tilted. Finally, in determining the axial length, one should clarify which particular axial length was employed, whether it was along the visual axis or along the orbital axis.

KARGER

Fax +41 61 306 12 34
E-Mail karger@karger.ch
www.karger.com

1661–3406/08/0052–0060$24.50/0

Accessible online at:
www.karger.com/nba

Dr. David T. Yew
Department of Anatomy
Chinese University of Hong Kong
Shatin, N.T., Hong Kong, SAR (China)
Tel. +852 2609 6899, Fax +852 2603 5031, E-Mail david-yew@cuhk.edu.hk

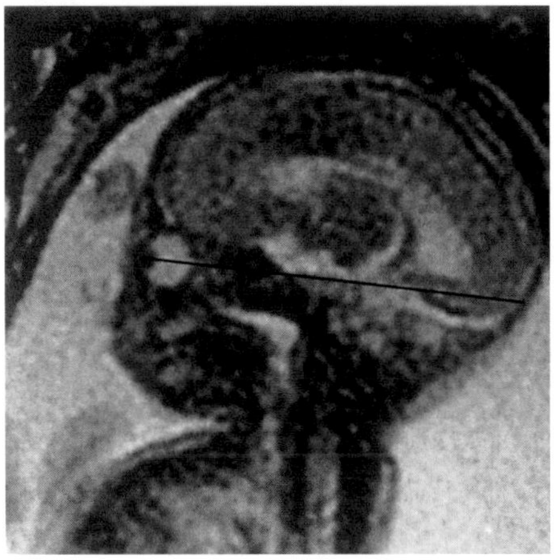

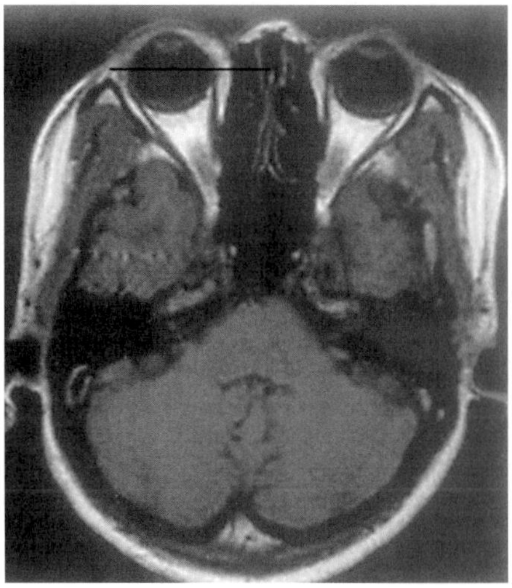

Fig. 1. Horizontal line measurements through the eye and from the cornea to the external occipital protuberance of the fetus in a parasagittal vertical MRI section. **Fig. 2.** The transverse line allowed measurements through the tip of the zygomatic bone to the median nasal septum of the fetus in a transverse MRI section, allowing also measurement of the transverse diameter of the eye.

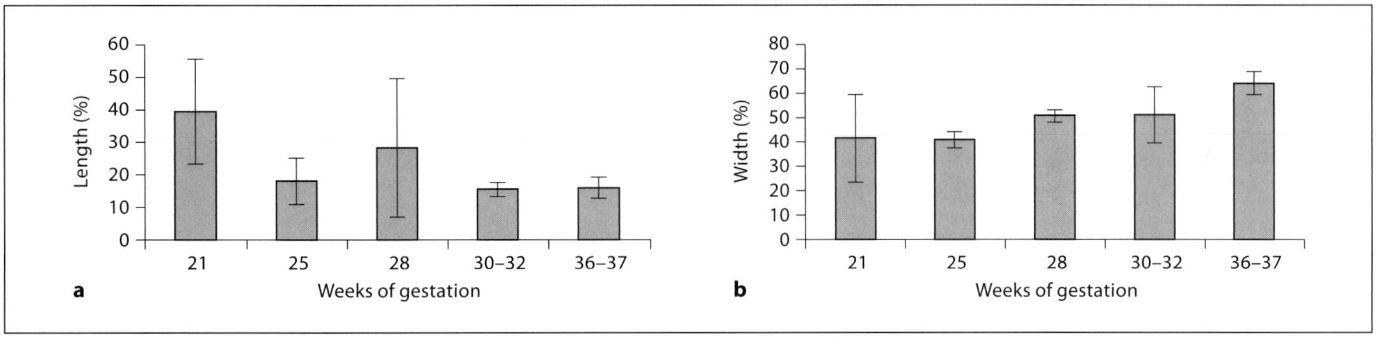

Fig. 3. a The proportion of the AP length of the eye versus the AP length from the mid cornea to the external occipital protuberance of the fetuses at different ages. **b** The proportion of the transverse diameter of the eye along the line of the tip of the zygomatic bone to the median septum of the fetuses of different ages.

Along this line of reasoning, we have therefore performed a small study utilizing 27 live fetuses at 21–37 weeks of gestation (4 of 21 weeks, 7 of 25–26 weeks, 4 of 28 weeks, 6 of 30–32 weeks and 6 of 36–37 weeks) of normal pregnant women who had consented to the imaging with the approval of the hospitals in Guangzhou and Kunming (Faculty of Medicine, Sun Yat Sen University, and Kunming Medical University). MR images were taken and analyzed.

MR Imaging

With the consent of the mothers and the ethical committees of the hospitals, the pregnant women with these live fetuses were scanned by MRI. MR imaging was performed in the affiliated hospitals of Medical Faculty of the Sun Yat Sen University and the Kunming Medical University, Kunming, China.

MR imaging was performed using a Signa Excite 1.5-tesla scanner (General Electric Medical System, Milwaukee, Wisc., USA) with shielded magnetic field gradients of up to 77 mT/ms and a four-channel body coin (TORSO-PA). When scanned, all the mothers held their breath. The following parameters were set (slice thickness = 5 mm, gap = 1 mm, field of view = 35 × 35). MRI were taken using a T_2-weighted single shot fast spin echo sequence (TR/TE = 800/80 ms, matrix = 384 × 224, bandwidth = 62.5 kHz, slice thickness/gap = 3 mm/0 mm, holding breath time = 10–20 s). All the mothers were placed supine and MRI started from the lower limb up.

Firstly, from the midparasagittal sections of these fetuses, a line was drawn from the mid cornea to the external occipital protuberance and the total length measured. Afterwards, the anteroposterior (AP) length from the mid cornea to the back of the eyeball along the same line was also measured (fig. 1). The latter measurements were expressed

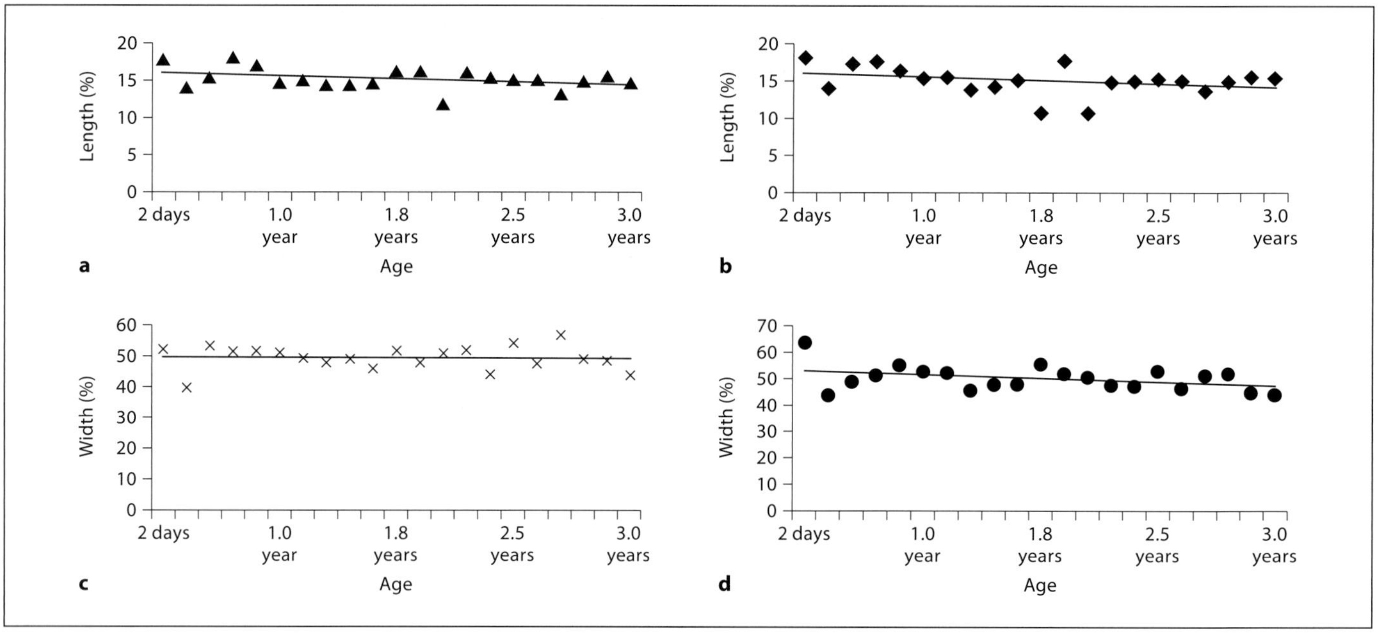

Fig. 4. **a**, **b** Percentage of the AP lengths of the right (**a**) and left eye (**b**) versus the AP length of the mid cornea to the external occipital protuberance of the same eye of the neonates up to 3 years of age. **c**, **d** Percentage of the transverse diameter of the right (**c**) and left eye (**d**) versus the diameter from the zygomatic bone to the nasal septum of the neonates up to 3 years of age.

as a percentage of the total (the corneal-occipital length). In addition to the fetuses, 21 neonatal infants ranging from 2 days to 3 years of age had been subjected to MRI and the same parameters were calculated as in the fetuses. All sections used for measurements were cut through the cornea and a major part of the lens of the eyes.

Secondly, using the transverse sections of MRI, a line was drawn through the tip of the zygomatic bone to the median nasal septum, passing through the eye transversely (fig. 2). The diameter through the eye (diameter) was expressed as a ratio of the zygomatic bone to the nasal septum along the same line. Again the sectional plane passed through the cornea and the major diameter of the lens.

The results obtained (fig. 3) indicated that the ratio of the AP lengths of the eyes in the fetuses actually decreased significantly from 28 weeks of gestation to term, projecting a higher cranial AP growth than the AP growth of the eye. On the other hand, in the fetus, the transverse diameter of the eye increased till term, i.e. the eyes were increasing in this dimension and represented an increasingly large portion of the growing face, i.e. eye diameter increases faster than the diameter of the face. From another angle, in the neonatal infant (fig. 4) ≤3 years of age, AP and transverse growth of the eye were horizontal and in fact showed somewhat decreasing trends, indicating the growth of the AP axial length and transverse diameters were not equivalent to the rapid lengthening or the transverse diameter increase in the head and face. Therefore, using different lines through the eye, e.g. through the orbital axis (the optic nerve), one could yet derive other more interesting conclusions for the growth of eye. This is a point that should be taken into consideration in future morphometric studies.

References

1 Denis D, Faure F, Volot F, Scheiner C, Boubli L, Dezard X, Saracco JB: Ocular growth in the fetus. 2. Comparative study of the growth of the globe and the orbit and the parameters of fetal growth. Ophthalmologica 1993;207:125–132.

2 Denis D, Righini M, Scheiner C, Volot F, Boubli L, Dezard X, Vola J, Saracco JB: Ocular growth in the fetus. 1. Comparative study of axial length and biometric parameters in the fetus. Ophthalmologica 1993;207:117–124.

3 Denis D, Burguière O, Burillon C: A biometric study of the eye, orbit, and face in 205 normal human fetuses. Invest Ophthalmol Vis Sci 1998;39:2232–2238.

4 Goldstein I, Tamir A, Zimmer EZ, Itskovitz-Eldor J: Growth of the fetal orbit and lens in normal pregnancies. Ultrasound Obstet Gynecol 1998;12:175–179.

5 Dilmen G, Köktener A, Turhan NO, Tez S: Growth of the fetal lens and orbit. Int J Gynaecol Obstet 2002;76:267–271.

6 Tomasik E, Czepita D, Zejmo M, Czerwiński F: Development of the human eyeball and orbit during the fetal life. Ann Acad Med Stetin 2005;51:37–40.

Neuroembryology and Aging

Neuroembryol Aging 2008;5:63–66
DOI: 10.1159/000116735

Received: July 17, 2007
Accepted: September 8, 2007
Published online: August 19, 2008

Use of Fluorescence Fundus Angiography to Assess Variations in Retinal Circulation in Myopic Patients of Different Ages

Xi Ying[a] Yan Wu[a] Yi Wang[a] Li Ran[a] David T. Yew[b]

[a]Department of Ophthalmology, Southwest Hospital, Third Military Medical University, Chongqing, and
[b]Department of Anatomy, Chinese University of Hong Kong, Hong Kong, SAR, China

Key Words
Age · Fluorescence · Fundus angiography · Myopia · Retinal circulation

Abstract
To investigate the variation in retinal circulation in patients with different degrees of myopia and different age by fluorescence fundus angiography (FFA). Thirty myopic patients (60 eyes), 20–54 years of age, with various degrees of myopia were evaluated. All patients underwent fundus photography and FFA using a standard technique. Patients with other ophthalmologic diseases possibly affecting the retrobulbar circulation and those with a history of laser treatment or intraocular surgery were excluded. Vascular filling patterns at arterial phase, arterial-venous phase and venous phase were reviewed. The average filling times at each phase were significantly delayed in severe myopia, but there was no difference between eyes with mild and medium myopia. There was no statistically significant correlation between mean filling time and age. The findings indicated a significant correlation between the intraocular blood circulation and the degree of myopia.

Introduction

Myopia is a common eye problem worldwide. Over the past decades, the prevalence rate of myopia has increased, reaching epidemic rates in the Asian population [1–3]. The age-old question of the roles of nature and nurture in this process remain unanswered. Twin studies of segregation analysis and association studies have demonstrated that hereditary factors play an important role in myopia development [4–7]. The data suggest that environmental factors might also interact with genetic factors to increase the risks of developing myopia [8, 9]. A severe degree of myopia increases the risk of developing sight-threatening ocular pathology, such as retinal degeneration and glaucoma [10, 11]. Further research is needed to elucidate the risks of developing myopia.

Fluorescence fundus angiography (FFA) is a routine technique that can be used to assess retinal circulation. Fluorescein, an inert vegetable dye, is injected into an arm vein and its passage through the retinal circulation is photographed using blue excitation illumination. The use of a low-light-level-sensitive, high-resolution, intensified video camera allows real-time recording of the retinal fluorescein angiograms. It is generally used to image lesions in diabetic retinopathy, retinal periphlebitis and uveitis, for example. FFA has also played a role in the clinical assessment of myopia. Recent studies have shown

KARGER

Fax +41 61 306 12 34
E-Mail karger@karger.ch
www.karger.com

1661–3496/08/0052–0063$24.50/0

Accessible online at:
www.karger.com/nba

Dr. David T. Yew
Department of Anatomy, Chinese University of Hong Kong
Shatin, N.T., Hong Kong, SAR (China)
Tel. +852 2609 6899, Fax +852 2603 5031, E-Mail david-yew@cuhk.edu.hk

that the pathologic changes in the posterior pole of the fundus appeared with different degrees of damage, e.g. simple, diffuse, psoriasis and complex lesions [12]. The higher the diopter (D), the greater the pathologic change at the fundus, and the more severe the level of damage. To assess blood flow in eye arteries in patients with myopia, Karczewicz and Modrzejewska [13] found that a statistically significant decrease in velocity correlated with the value of refractive error using Doppler ultrasonography. Furthermore, the choroidal, retinal and intracranial circulation has been decreased in degenerative myopia using color Doppler imaging [14, 15]. The choroidal vasculature may be significantly altered in highly myopic eyes, being more prevalent in eyes with posterior staphyloma (backward bulging of the sclera at the posterior pole of the eye) [16]. However, to our knowledge, there have been no reports on the retinal circulation in myopic patients at different filling phases.

In this work, we aimed to investigate the variations in the retinal circulation and the filling times in the arterial, arterial-venous and venous phases in patients with various degrees of myopia. A retrospective investigation of FFAs performed in patients with myopic degeneration was conducted.

Patients and Methods

FFAs and medical records of 30 myopic patients (60 eyes) with various degrees of myopia were evaluated. The patients had all been examined at the Southwest Hospital, Chongqing, from January 2003 until June 2007. Ethical consent for the use of these medical records was obtained from the Hospital Authority of the Southwest Hospital, Chongqing. Of these patients, 13 were male and 17 were female. Ages ranged from 20 to 54 years, with a mean of 34.52 years. Twenty-five (41.7%) eyes ranged from –0.25 to –3.00 D (mild myopia), 18 eyes (30%) from –3.00 to –6.00 D (medium myopia) and 17 eyes (28.3%) <–6.00 D (severe myopia). A complete ocular examination was conducted in all subjects including measurement of best-corrected visual acuity, slit lamp examination and intraocular pressure examination. All patients underwent fundus photography and FFA using a standard technique. Patients with other ophthalmologic diseases possibly affecting the retrobulbar circulation, such as diabetic retinopathy, hypertensive retinopathy, age-related maculopathy, glaucoma, and those with a history of laser treatment or intraocular surgery, were excluded.

Vascular filling patterns were reviewed. Angiographic evidence was based on the filling time at the arterial, arterial-venous and venous phases. We excluded all cases that were markedly out of focus or had equivocal continuity of vascular filling.

All data were analyzed using paired t tests. Data were presented as means ± SD. p values < 0.05 were considered significant.

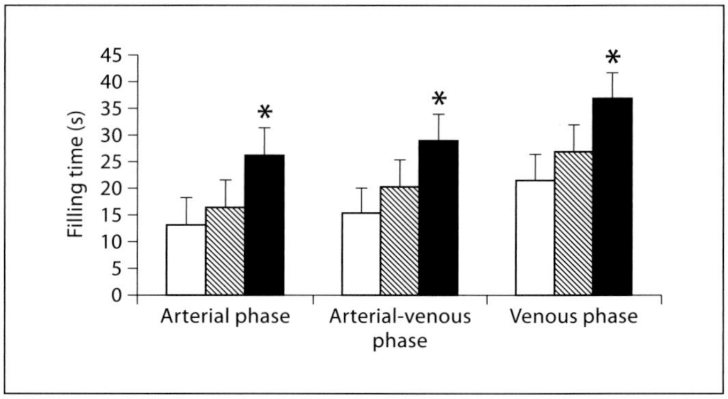

Fig. 1. Filling times at different vascular filling patterns of myopia. * $p < 0.05$. □ = mild myopia; ▨ = medium myopia; ■ = severe myopia.

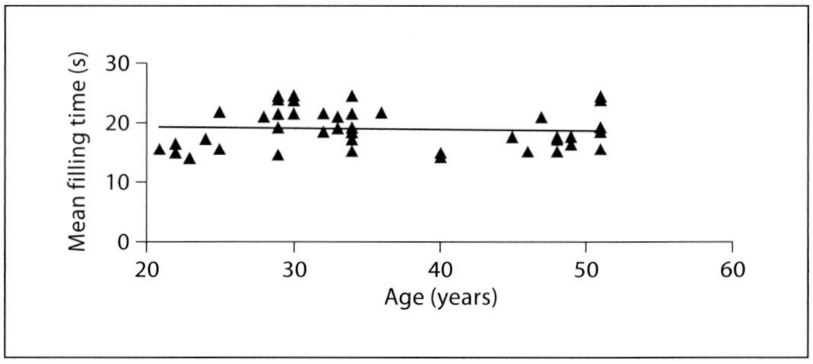

Fig. 2. Correlation between mean filling time and age in mild and medium myopic eyes ($r = 0.041$, $p > 0.05$).

Results

The FFA filling time measurements were summarized in figure 1. The average filling times in the arterial phase in mild, medium and severe myopia were 13.2 ± 2.59, 16.6 ± 1.82 and 26.2 ± 2.77 s, respectively. There was no difference between mild and medium myopia but a significant delay in severe myopia. At the arterial-venous phase, the mean filling times were 15.2 ± 3.27, 20.4 ± 2.88 and 28.8 ± 3.11 s, respectively, in mild, medium and severe myopic eyes. At the venous phase, mean filling times in mild and medium myopia were 21.4 ± 2.07 and 27 ± 3.54 s, respectively, versus 36.8 ± 4.15 s in the severe myopic eyes. The FFA filling time delay was most obvious in severe myopia, but there was no significant difference between mild and moderate myopia.

Using linear regression analysis, no statistically significant correlation between mean filling time and age was found in the mild and moderate myopic eyes ($r = 0.041$; $p > 0.05$; fig. 2).

Discussion

In the present study, a significant correlation between the intraocular blood circulation and the degrees of myopia was found. Also, the average retinal filling time was significantly delayed in severe myopic eyes. These results were in agreement with a previous color Doppler imaging study that measured obviously decreased velocity in the posterior ciliary and central retinal arteries in patients with degenerative myopia [17, 18]. Our results were also coherent with a study that revealed longer circulatory transit times in patients with high and complicated myopia compared to low and moderate myopia, suggesting a significant decrease in retinal circulation in severe myopia [19]. Circulatory abnormalities had also been found in other ophthalmologic disorders, e.g. age-related maculopathy [20, 21] and primary open-angle glaucoma [22–24]. More evidence has suggested that an increasing prevalence of primary open-angle glaucoma is related to the degree of myopia, with relatively greater risks for moderate and severe myopia compared to mild myopia [25–28]. Thus it is obviously important to investigate the circulation in ophthalmologic disorders.

A number of pathohistological studies have demonstrated smaller calibers of choroidal arteries, straightening of the retinal vessels, and thinning and loss of choriocapillaris capillaries in degenerative myopia [29–31]. These abnormalities might be associated with circulatory irregularities. In severe myopic eyes, the increase in ocular axial length causes stretching of scleral, choroidal and retinal tissue. These studies concluded that the need for oxygen and blood circulation declined due to atrophy of the choroidal and retinal tissue. In the present study, in each phase the filling time was significantly delayed in severe myopia compared with mild and medium myopic eyes. Previous studies reported that blood flow decreased in chicks with ocular enlargement due either to a decrease in local perfusion pressure or an increase in vascular resistivity [32]. Furthermore, in progressive myopic patients, the use of pentoxifylline, a drug that lowers blood viscosity and improves erythrocyte flexibility, significantly increased peak-systolic and end-diastolic flow velocities in the central retinal artery and short posterior ciliary arteries while resistance indices and systolic/diastolic ratios decreased [33]. These findings suggest that vascular dysfunction plays a key role in the development of myopia.

The data suggest that the filling time in the myopic eyes does not vary much with age. As several other studies had shown, pulsatile ocular blood flow decreased with increasing axial length in normal subjects. The axial length was a major factor affecting choroidal blood flow [34, 35]. However, myopic patients aged >60 years were not analyzed in present study.

In conclusion, using FFA, retinal filling times were significantly delayed at the arterial, arterial-venous and venous phases in severe myopic eyes, but apparently age neither affected nor correlated with this phenomenon. Measures to improve retinal circulation may be helpful to prevent the development of myopic complications.

References

1 Saw SM: A synopsis of the prevalence rates and environmental risk factors for myopia. Clin Exp Optom 2003;86:289–294.
2 Park DJ, Congdon NG: Evidence for an 'epidemic' of myopia. Ann Acad Med Singapore 2004;33:21–26.
3 Woo WW, Lim KA, Yang H, Lim XY, Liew F, Lee YS, Saw SM: Refractive errors in medical students in Singapore. Singapore Med J 2004; 45:470–474.
4 Tocyap ML, Azar N, Chen T, Wiggs J: Clinical and molecular characterization of a patient with an interstitial deletion of chromosome 12q15-q23 and peripheral corneal abnormalities. Am J Ophthalmol 2006;141: 566–567.
5 Jacobi FK, Zrenner E, Broghammer M, Pusch CM: A genetic perspective on myopia. Cell Mol Life Sci 2005;62:800–808.
6 Dirani M, Chamberlain M, Shekar SN, Islam AF, Garoufalis P, Chen CY, Guymer RH, Baird PN: Heritability of refractive error and ocular biometrics: the Genes in Myopia (GEM) twin study. Invest Ophthalmol Vis Sci 2006;47:4756–4761.
7 Yeh LK, Chiu CJ, Fong CF, Wang IJ, Chen WL, Hsiao CK, Huang SC, Shih YF, Hu FR, Lin LL: The genetic effect on refractive error and anterior corneal aberration: twin eye study. J Refract Surg 2007;23:257–265.
8 Chen CY, Scurrah KJ, Stankovich J, Garoufalis P, Dirani M, Pertile KK, Richardson AJ, Mitchell P, Baird PN: Heritability and shared environment estimates for myopia and associated ocular biometric traits: the Genes in Myopia (GEM) family study. Hum Genet 2007;121:511–520.
9 Feldkämper M, Schaeffel F: Interactions of genes and environment in myopia. Dev Ophthalmol 2003;37:34–49.
10 Yap M, Cho J, Woo G: A survey of low vision patients in Hong Kong. Clin Exp Optom 1990;73:19–22.
11 Seet B, Wong TY, Tan DT, Saw SM, Balakrishnan V, Lee LK, Lim AS: Myopia in Singapore: taking a public health approach. Br J Ophthalmol 2001;85:521–526.
12 Yu R: Affection of diopters and fundus pathologic changes in high myopic eyes (in Chinese). Yan Ke Xue Bao 2003;19:211–214.
13 Karczewicz D, Modrzejewska M: Blood flow in eye arteries assessed by Doppler ultrasound in patients with myopia (in Polish). Klin Oczna 2004;106:211–213.
14 Akyol N, Kükner AS, Ozdemir T, Esmerligil S: Choroidal and retinal blood flow changes in degenerative myopia. Can J Ophthalmol 1996;31:113–119.

15 Dolzhich GI, Nidal Abed AKh: The relationship of the indices of intracranial collateral circulation to variants in the clinical course of acquired high myopia (in Russian). Vestn Oftalmol 1999;115:23–25.
16 Moriyama M, Ohno-Matsui K, Futagami S, Yoshida T, Hayashi K, Shimada N, Kojima A, Tokoro T, Mochizuki M: Morphology and long-term changes of choroidal vascular structure in highly myopic eyes with and without posterior staphyloma. Ophthalmology 2007;114:1755–1762.
17 Shimada N, Ohno-Matsui K, Harino S, Yoshida T, Yasuzumi K, Kojima A, Kobayashi K, Futagami S, Tokoro T, Mochizuki M: Reduction of retinal blood flow in high myopia. Graefes Arch Clin Exp Ophthalmol 2004; 242:284–288.
18 Dimitrova G, Tamaki Y, Kato S, Nagahara M: Retrobulbar circulation in myopic patients with or without myopic choroidal neovascularisation. Br J Ophthalmol 2002;86: 771–773.
19 Avetisov ES, Savitskaya NF: Some features of ocular microcirculation in myopia. Ann Ophthalmol 1977;9:1261–1264.
20 Remulla JF, Gaudio AR, Miller S, Sandberg MA: Foveal electroretinograms and choroidal perfusion characteristics in fellow eyes of patients with unilateral neovascular age-related macular degeneration. Br J Ophthalmol 1995;79:558–561.
21 Ciulla TA, Harris A, Chung HS, Danis RP, Kagemann L, McNulty L, Pratt LM, Martin BJ: Color Doppler imaging discloses reduced ocular blood flow velocities in nonexudative age-related macular degeneration. Am J Ophthalmol 1999;128:75–80.
22 Delaney Y, Walshe TE, O'Brien C: Vasospasm in glaucoma: clinical and laboratory aspects. Optom Vis Sci 2006;83:406–414.
23 Grieshaber MC, Flammer J: Blood flow in glaucoma. Curr Opin Ophthalmol 2005;16: 79–83.
24 Gherghel D, Hosking SL, Cunliffe IA: Abnormal systemic and ocular vascular response to temperature provocation in primary open-angle glaucoma patients: a case for autonomic failure? Invest Ophthalmol Vis Sci 2004;45:3546–3554.
25 Németh J, Michelson G, Harazny J: Retinal microcirculation correlates with ocular wall thickness, axial eye length, and refraction in glaucoma patients. J Glaucoma 2001;10:390–395.
26 Dolzhich GI, Shlyk IV, Dolzhich RR: Clinical variants of glaucoma in patients with acquired high myopia (in Russian). Vestn Oftalmol 1999;115:3–6.
27 Karczewicz D, Modrzejewska M: Assessment of blood flow in eye arteries in patients with myopia and glaucoma (in Polish). Klin Oczna 2004;106:214–216.
28 Loyo-Berríos NI, Blustein JN: Primary-open glaucoma and myopia: a narrative review. WMJ 2007;106:85–89.
29 Ohno-Matsui K, Morishima N, Ito M, Yamashita S, Futagami S, Tokoro T, Nakagawa T: Indocyanine green angiography of retrobulbar vascular structures in severe myopia. Am J Ophthalmol 1997;123:494–505.
30 Quaranta M, Arnold J, Coscas G, Français C, Quentel G, Kuhn D, Soubrane G: Indocyanine green angiographic features of pathologic myopia. Am J Ophthalmol 1996;122: 663–671.
31 Hirata A, Negi A: Morphological changes of choriocapillaris in experimentally induced chick myopia. Graefes Arch Clin Exp Ophthalmol 1998;236:132–137.
32 Shih YF, Fitzgerald MEC, Reiner A: Choroidal blood flow is reduced in chicks with ocular enlargement induced by corneal incisions. Curr Eye Res 1993;12:229–237.
33 Urban B, Ustymowicz A, Bakunowicz-Lazarczyk A, Kretowska M: Effect of pentoxifylline on Doppler blood flow parameters in the central retinal artery and the short posterior ciliary arteries in adolescents with progressive myopia (in Polish). Klin Oczna 2004;106:318–320.
34 Mori F, Konno S, Hikichi T, Yamaguchi Y, Ishiko S, Yoshida A: Factors affecting pulsatile ocular blood flow in normal subjects. Br J Ophthalmol 2001;85:529–530.
35 Lam AK, Wong S, Lam CS, To CH: The effect of myopic axial elongation and posture on the pulsatile ocular blood flow in young normal subjects. Optom Vis Sci 2002;79:300–305.

Author Index Vol. 5, No. 1–2, 2008

Neuroembryology and Aging

KARGER

Fax +41 61 306 12 34
E-Mail karger@karger.ch
www.karger.com

Accessible online at:
www.karger.com/nba

Subject Index Vol. 5, No. 1–2, 2008

Neuroembryology and Aging

KARGER

Fax +41 61 306 12 34
E-Mail karger@karger.ch
www.karger.com

Accessible online at:
www.karger.com/nba